My
Kindergarten
Reading
Workbook

This book belongs to:

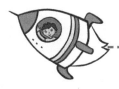

Way to Go!

After completing each activity, color a star to track how much you've done!

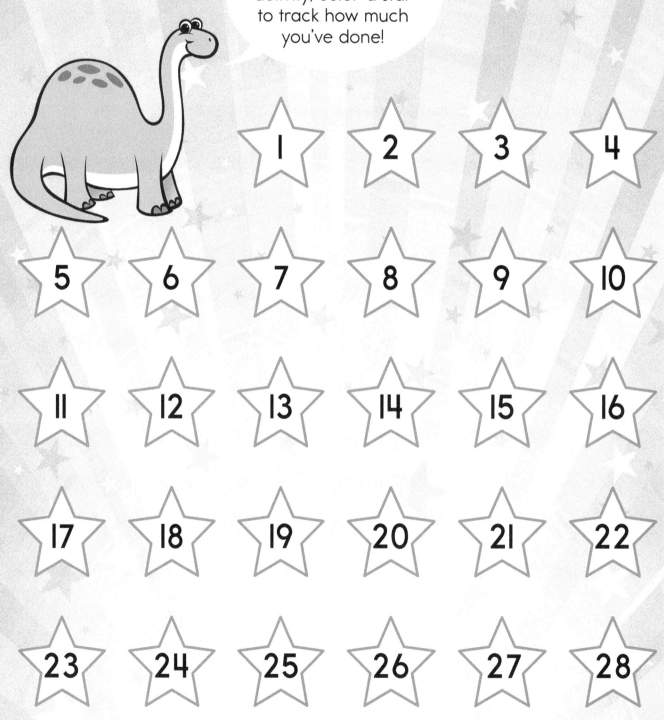

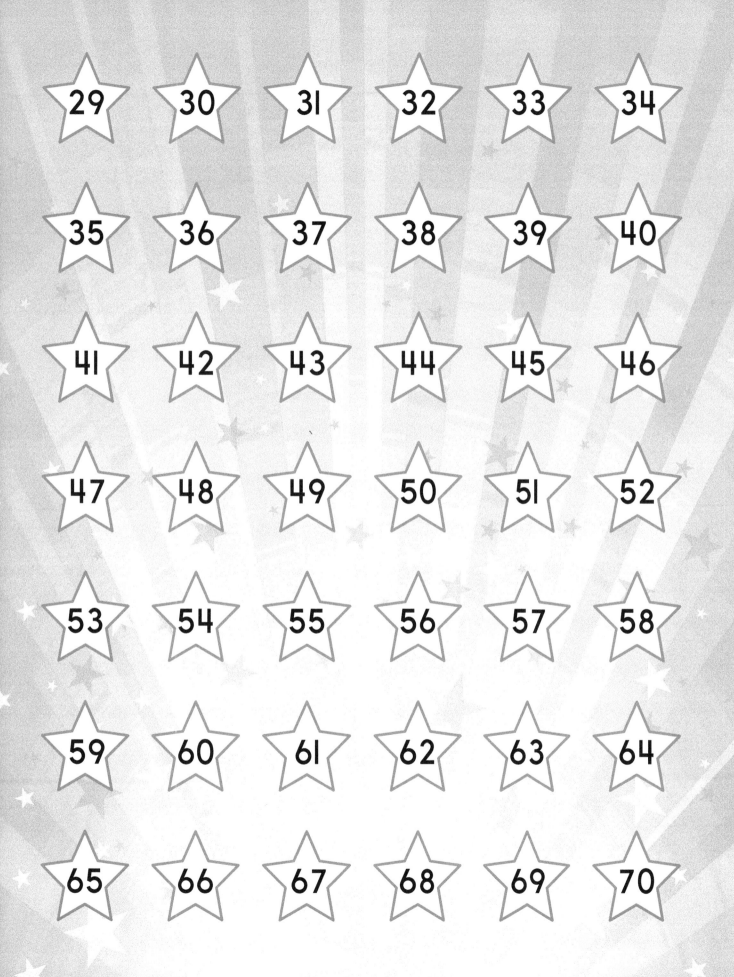

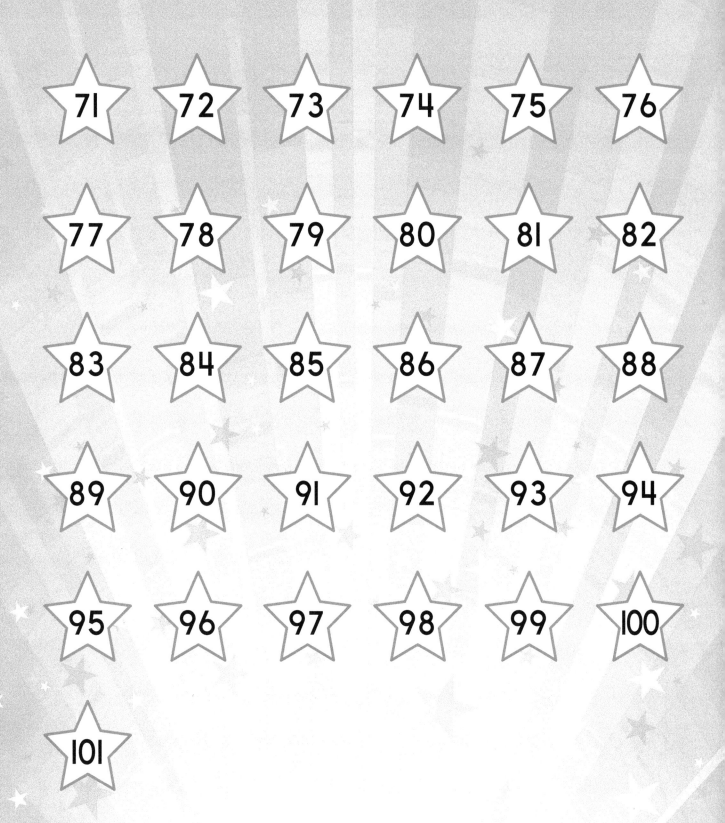

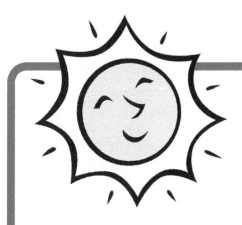

My

Kindergarten Reading Workbook

101 Games and Activities to Support Phonics and Sight Words

KIMBERLY ANN KIEDROWSKI

Illustrations by Robin Boyer

ROCKRIDGE
PRESS

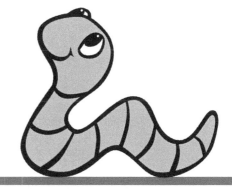

For general information on our other products and services or to obtain technical support, please contact our Customer Care Department within the United States at (866) 744-2665, or outside the United States at (510) 253-0500.

Rockridge Press publishes its books in a variety of electronic and print formats. Some content that appears in print may not be available in electronic books, and vice versa.

Series Designers: Stephanie Sumulong and Liz Cosgrove
Interior and Cover Designer: Scott Petrower
Art Producer: Megan Baggott
Editor: Alyson Penn
Production Editor: Nora Milman

Illustration © 2020-21 Robin Boyer

ISBN: Print 978-1-64739-162-1
R0

Contents

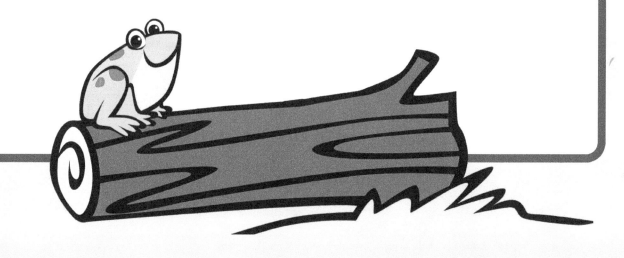

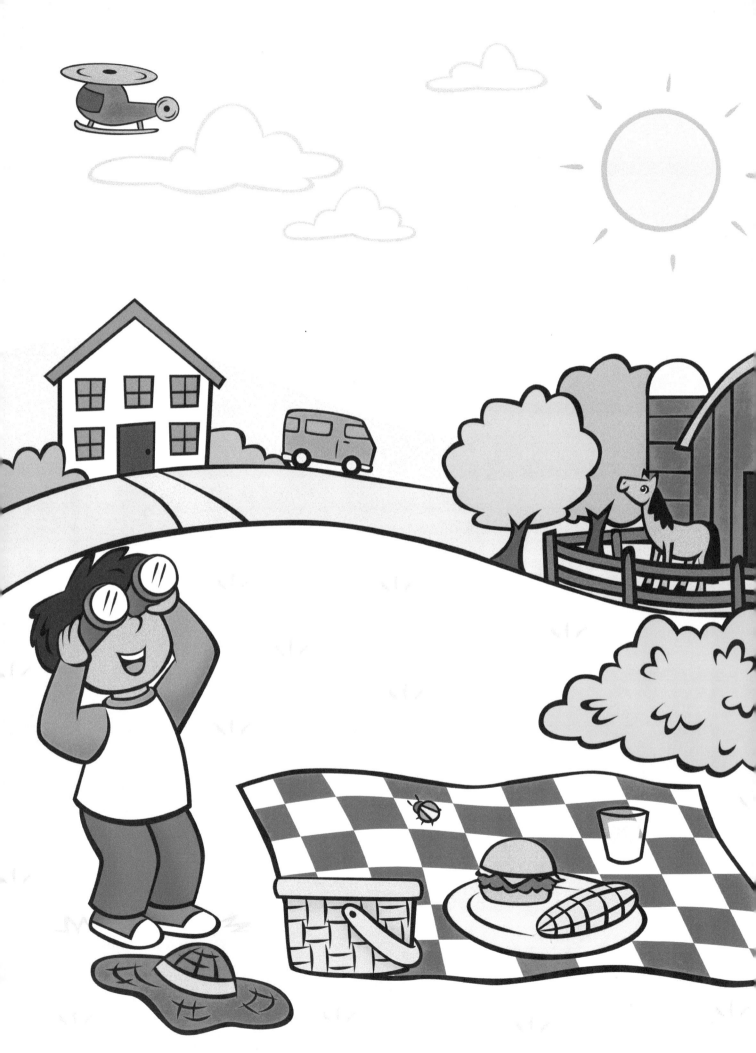

Note to Parents

Dear Parents,

Welcome to *My Kindergarten Reading Workbook*! Kindergarten is such a magical time, which begins with your child gaining the skills they need to become a successful reader. In this workbook, they will get a chance to practice these skills in a fun way!

The activities in the book are designed for children ages 5 to 6 and gradually increase in difficulty. Your kindergartner will start with the alphabet and move on to phonics skills that connect letters to sounds and words. Next, they will learn to read and write some of the words most frequently used in print with sight-word activities. The book will end by building upon these concepts with reading comprehension. By engaging your child with coloring, drawing, puzzles, and more, this book will help them gain confidence in their reading skills!

Each section of the book is color coded and progresses in a smooth learning pattern. Start each activity by reading the directions with your child, and let them work as best they can. Every child learns at a different pace. If your child begins to struggle with an activity, praise them for their effort and offer your help. Ideally, they should feel excited and motivated as they go through the book.

I hope that you and your child enjoy your time together with this workbook and that it will enhance your kindergartner's reading skills. Let the fun begin!

Kimberly

I. Pick the Apples

Draw a line from each apple to the matching basket.

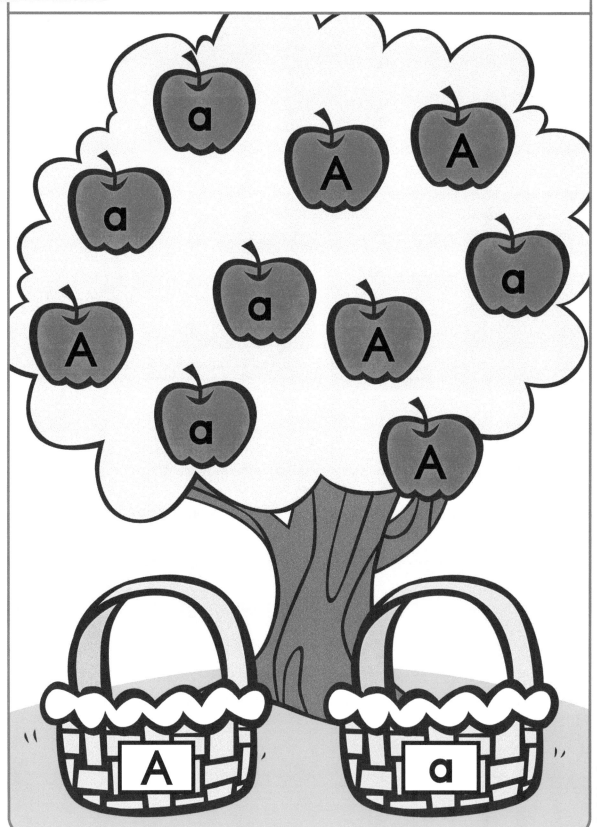

2. Day at the Beach

Circle each **B** and **b** hidden in the picture.

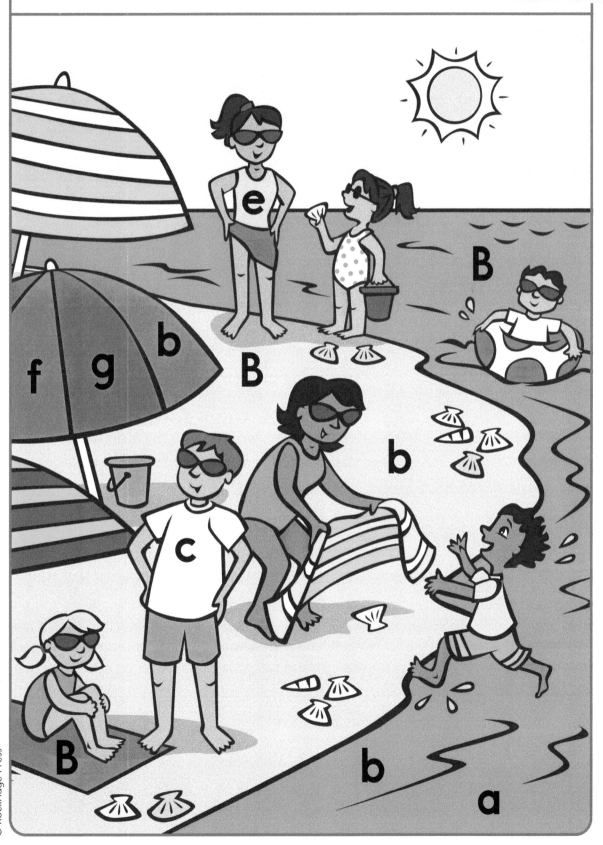

3. Come Home, Callie!

Help Callie Cat find her way home for dinner.
Follow **C** and **c** to get through the maze.

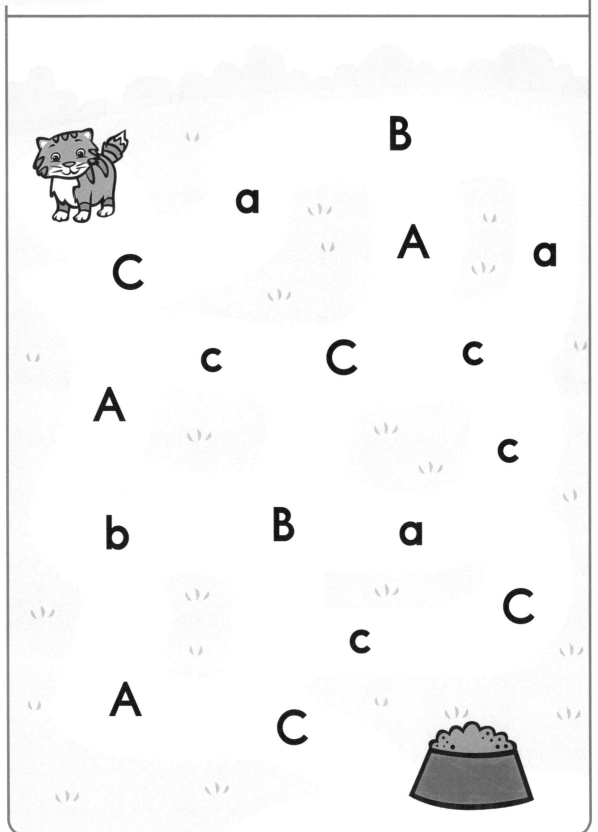

My Kindergarten Reading Workbook

© Rockridge Press

4. Dig It Up

Find the objects that begin with the letter **D** and color them.

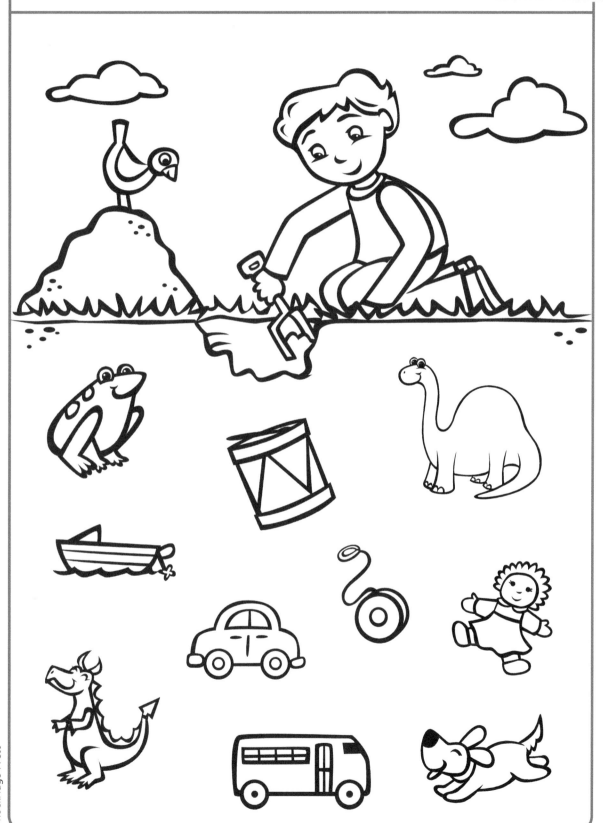

5. Letter Surprise

Color each space with the letter **E** gray. Color each space with **e** blue. What animal do you see?

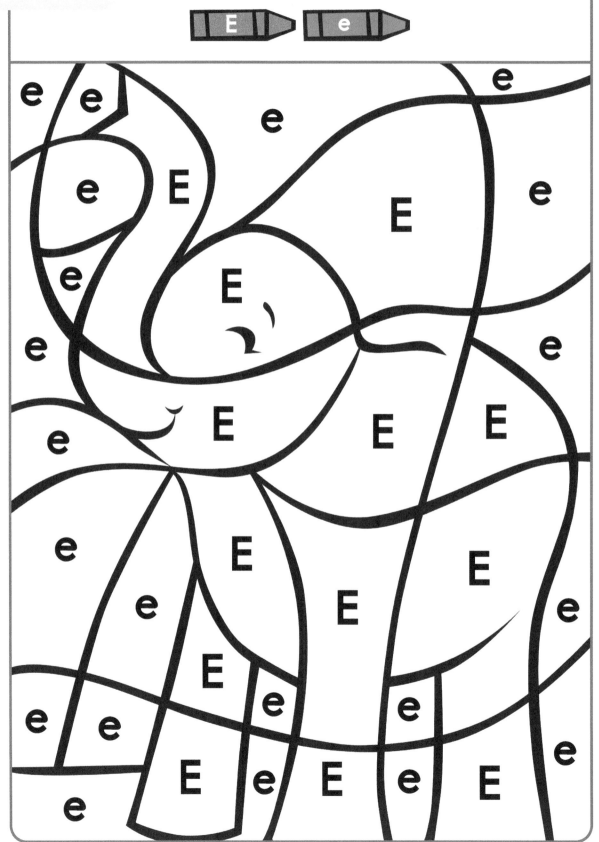

6. What Starts with F?

Draw a line to match each word to its picture.

fish

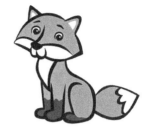

frog

fire

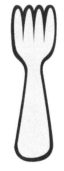

fox

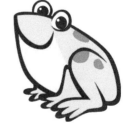

fork

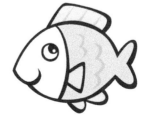

7. Fruity Fun

Connect the dots from **A** to **G**. What fruit did you find? Color the picture when you are finished.

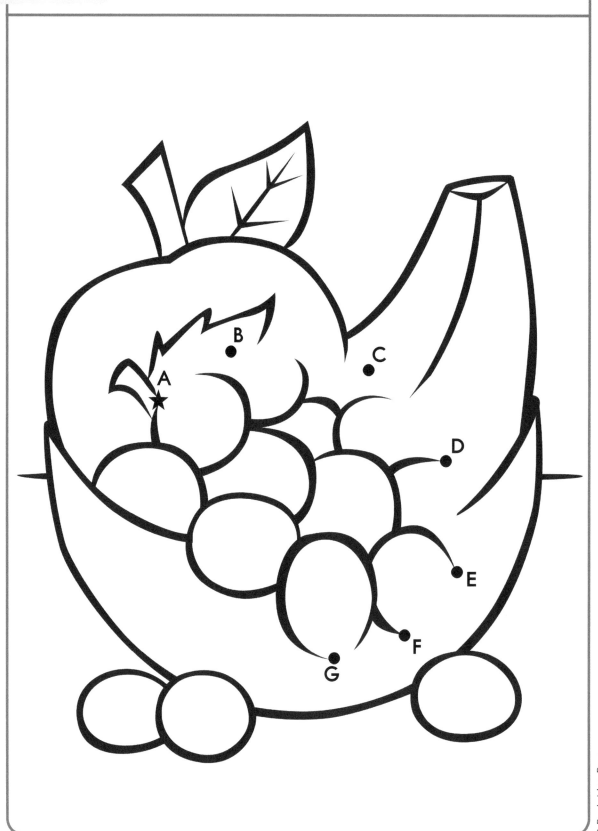

My Kindergarten Reading Workbook

8. Hippo Search

Find and circle each word hidden in the puzzle.

h	a	m	m	e	r	f	c
t	w	v	l	x	f	h	o
c	q	h	k	s	c	o	o
v	c	e	n	a	g	u	v
b	h	a	n	d	h	s	w
h	k	r	f	q	y	e	z
j	i	t	y	s	r	w	c
k	o	p	u	e	h	u	g

Word Bank

heart
hand
house
hug
hammer

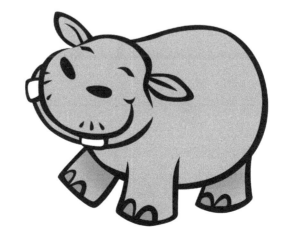

9. Ice Cream for Izzy

Izzy Penguin wants an ice cream cone! Follow **I** and **i** to help her through the maze.

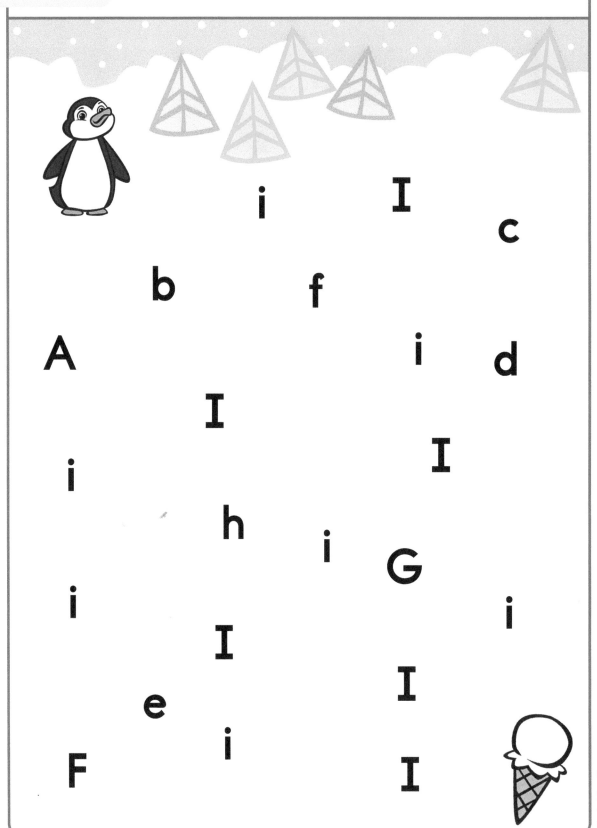

My Kindergarten Reading Workbook

10. In the Jungle

Circle each **J** and **j** hidden in the picture.

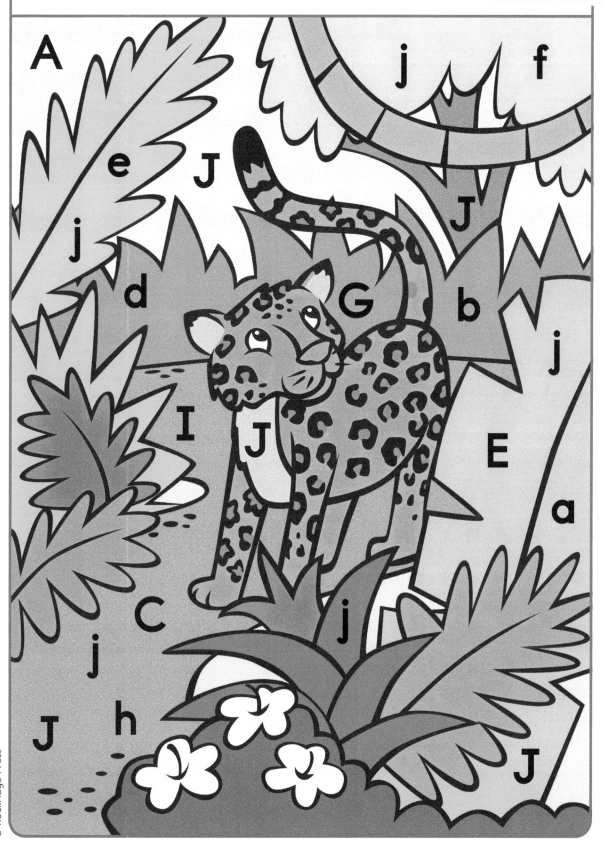

11. Fly a Kite

Color the picture below to fly a kite. Color the **K** spaces blue and the **k** spaces red.

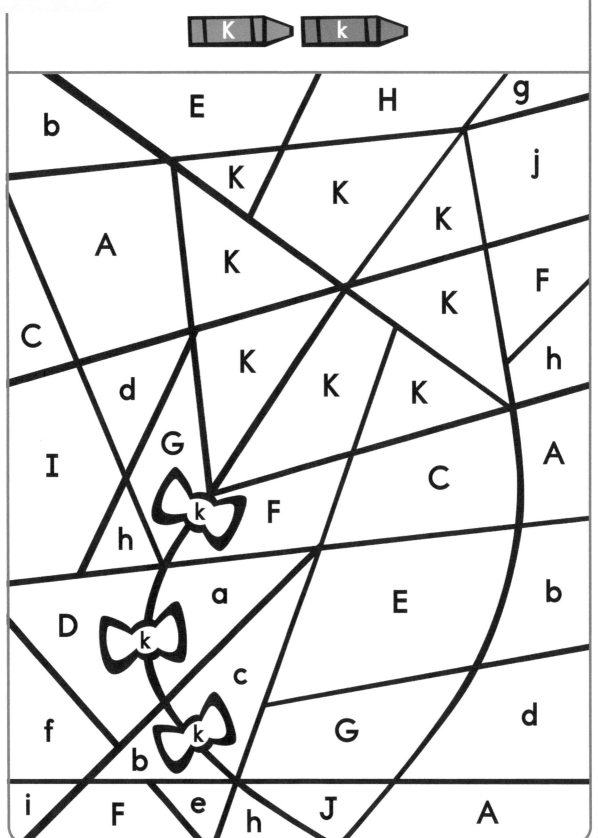

My Kindergarten Reading Workbook

12. Look for L!

Get **3** in a row by circling the pictures that begin with the letter **L**!

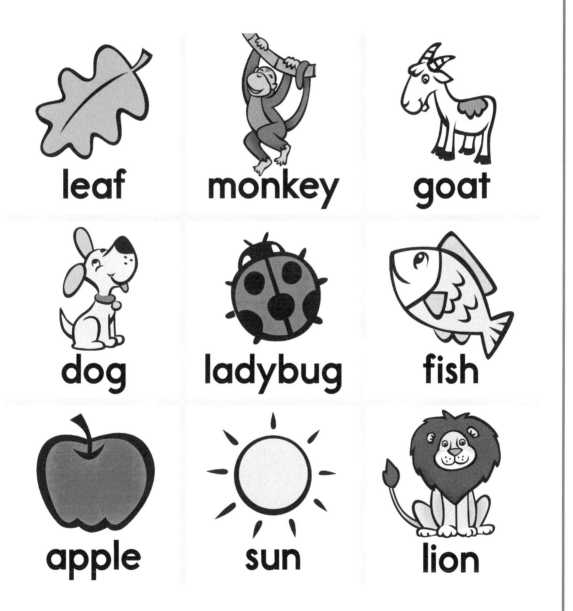

leaf   monkey   goat

dog   ladybug   fish

apple   sun   lion

13. Hang Around

Help Mia Monkey fill in the missing letters in the crossword puzzle.

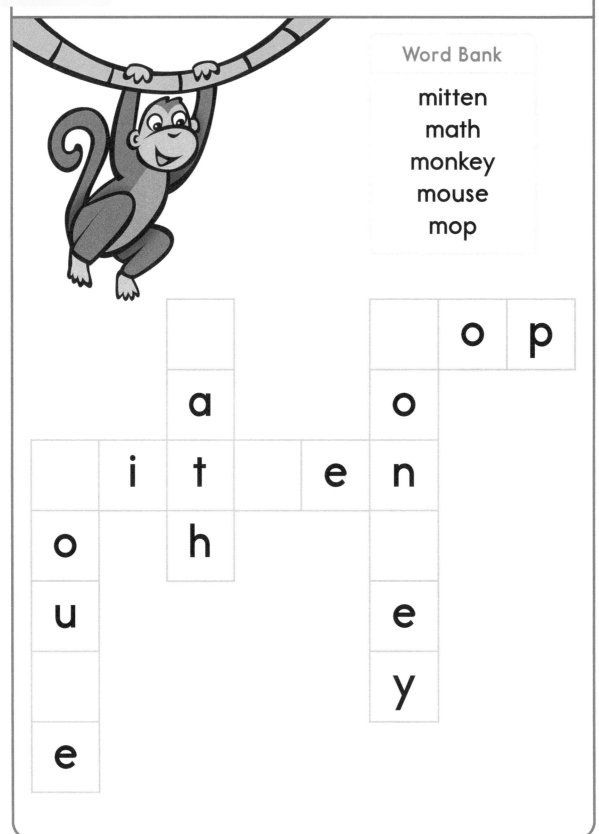

Word Bank

mitten
math
monkey
mouse
mop

14. Build a Nest

Connect the dots from **A** to **N** to make a nest! Say each letter out loud as you connect it. Color the picture when you are finished.

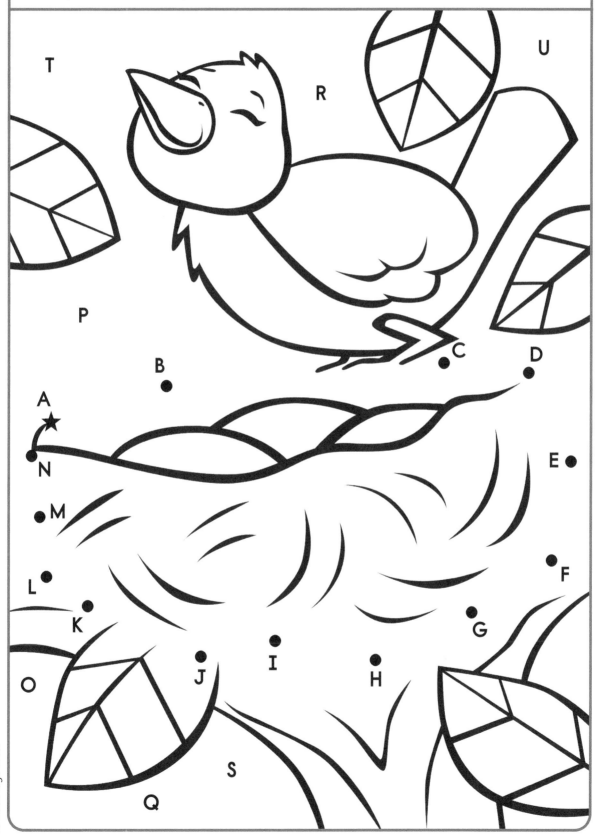

15. Out of this World

Ollie Alien is looking for objects that start with the letter **O**. Find and circle each one.

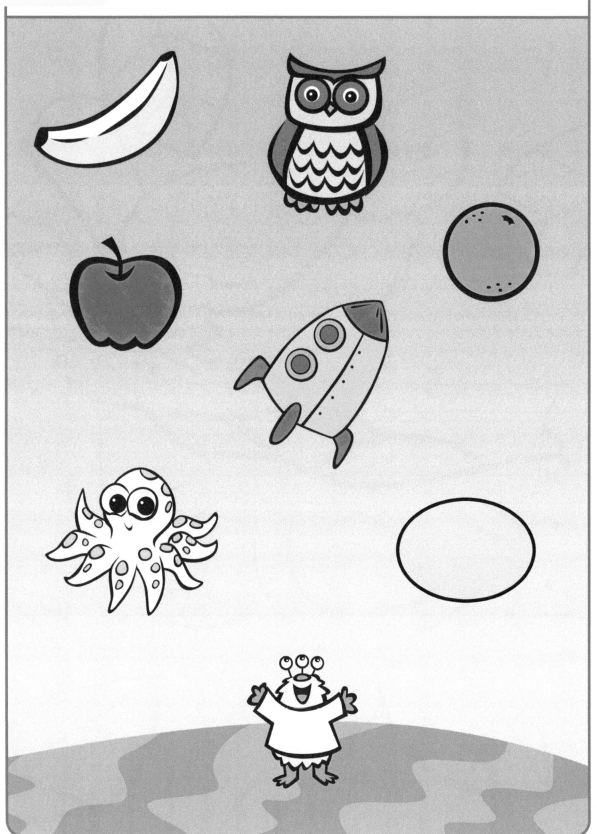

16. P is for . . .

Color the pictures that begin with the letter **P**!
Can you get **3** in a row?

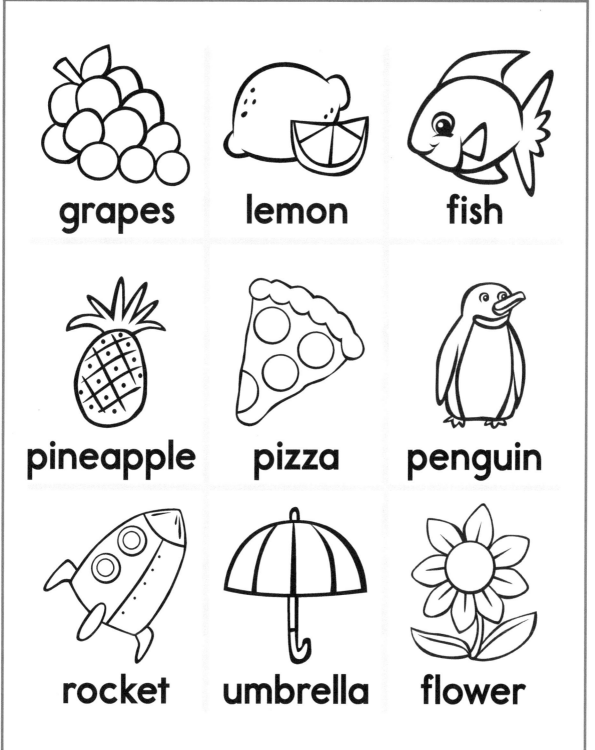

grapes   lemon   fish

pineapple   pizza   penguin

rocket   umbrella   flower

17. Castle Quest

Follow **Q** and **q** to help the knight get to the castle!

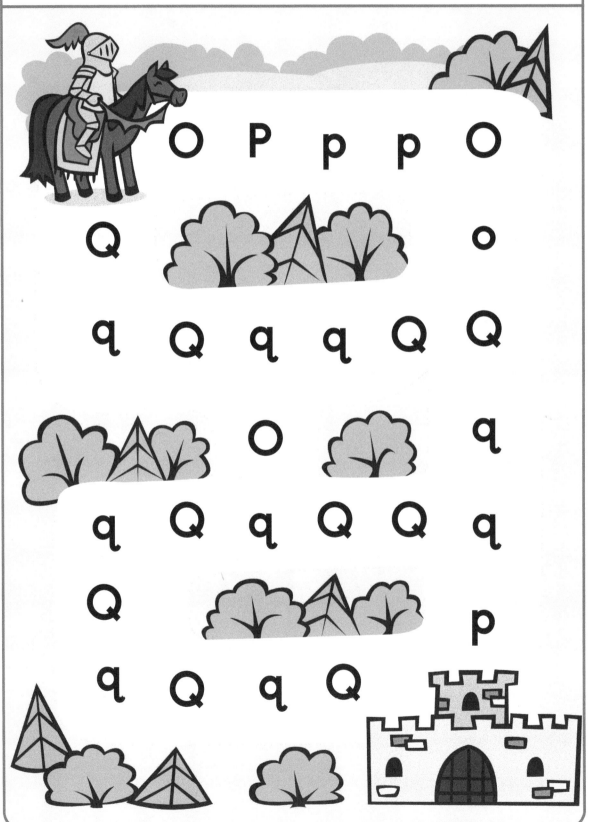

18. In My Room

Find and circle each object that begins with the letter **R**.

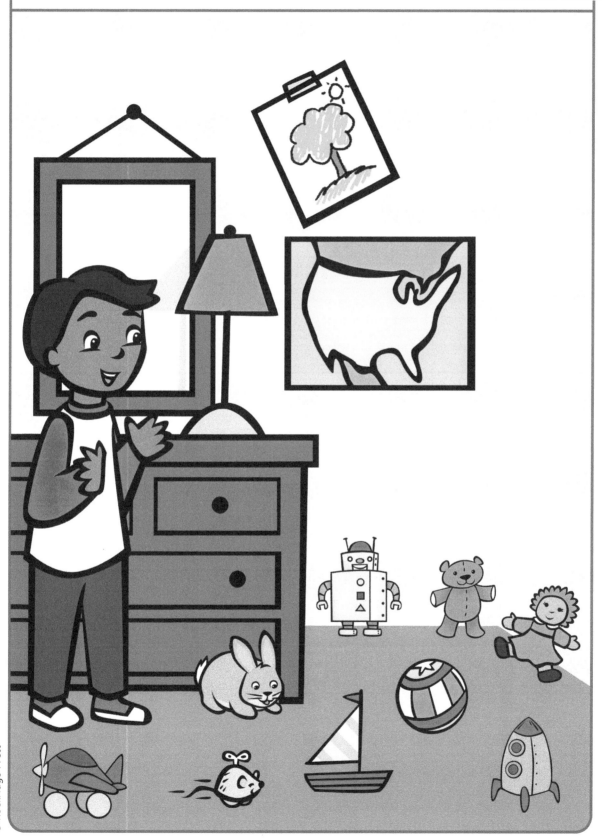

19. Silly Scramble

Unscramble the letters and write each word.
The pictures will give you a hint.

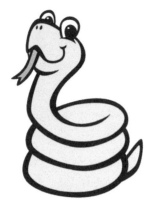

nakse

s

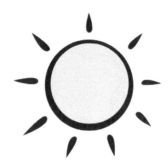

nus

s

arst

s

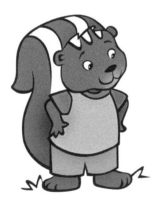

kunks

s

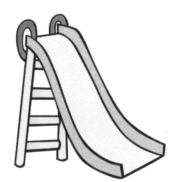

idesl

s

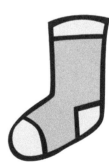

ocks

s

20. Time to Camp

The stars are shining! Draw a line from each **T** and **t** to the matching tent.

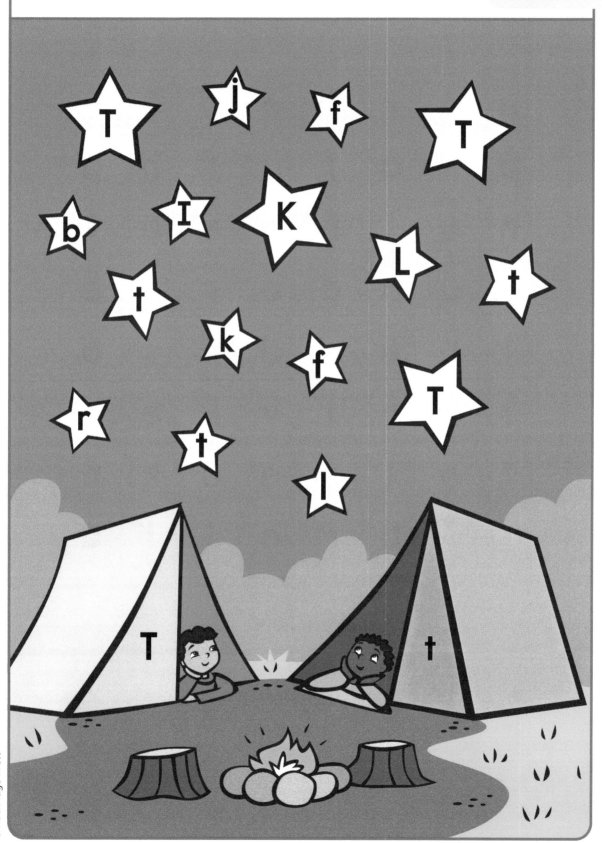

21. Under the Sea

Dive in to find and circle all the words that start with the letter **U**.

u	a	r	m	e	r	f	u
p	w	a	l	u	f	h	n
h	q	i	k	p	c	o	i
i	u	n	d	e	r	u	c
l	h	a	o	d	h	s	o
l	k	r	l	y	k	e	r
t	n	l	p	e	o	k	n
u	m	b	r	e	l	l	a

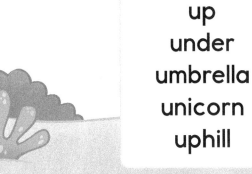

Word Bank

up
under
umbrella
unicorn
uphill

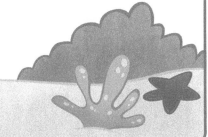

22. Sweet Music

Connect the dots from **A** to **V** to discover the musical instrument! Color the picture when you are finished.

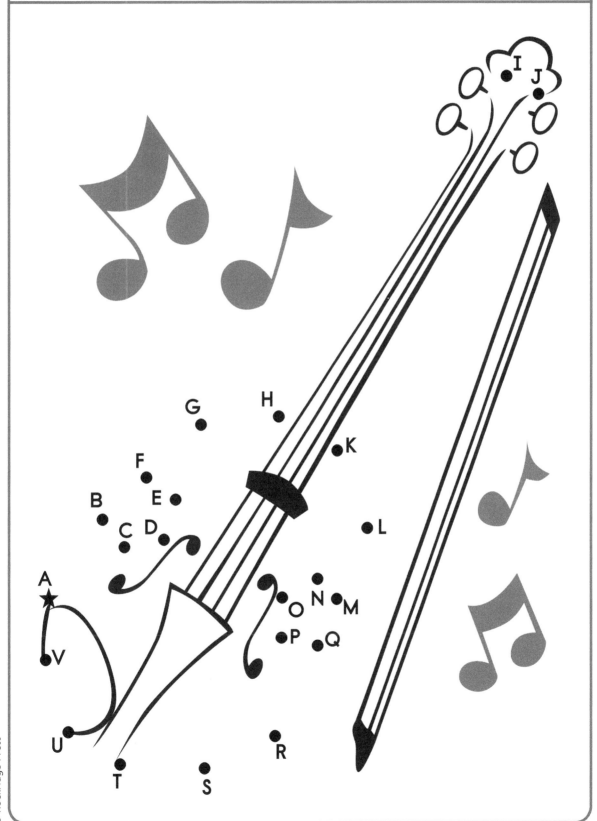

23. Where Is W?

Color the pictures that begin with the letter **W**.
Three in a row makes tic-tac-toe!

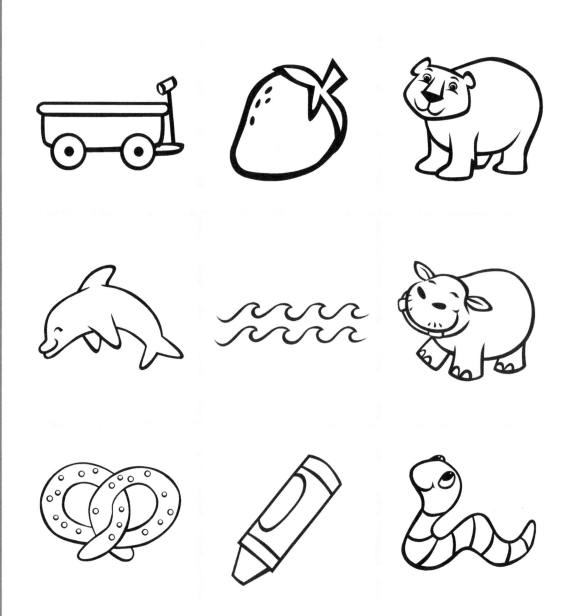

My Kindergarten Reading Workbook

24. X Marks the Spot

Color the letters on the map. Color **x** spaces **brown**.
Color the rest of the letters **blue**.

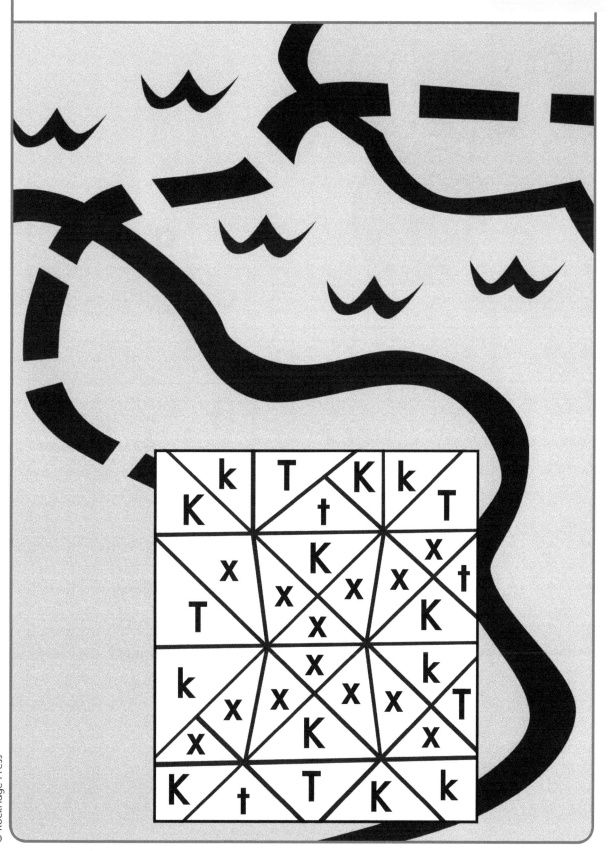

25. Yo-Yo Puzzle

Fill in the missing letters of each word in the puzzle.

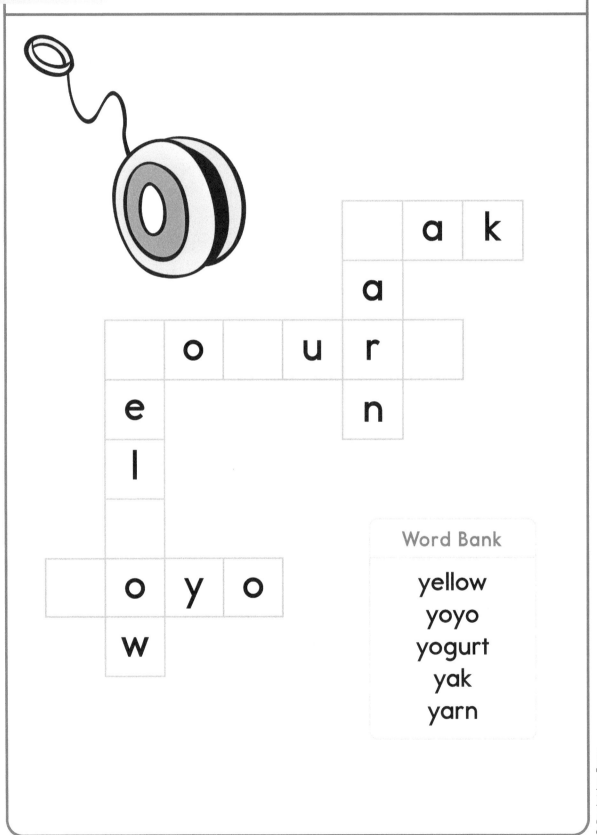

			a	k
		a		
o		u	r	
			n	

e
l
o y o
w

Word Bank

yellow
yoyo
yogurt
yak
yarn

© Rockridge Press

26. Missing Z!

The words are missing letters! Write each letter, say the word, and match its picture.

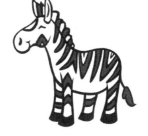

_zero

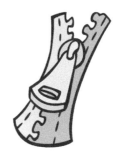

_o_

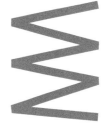

_eb_a

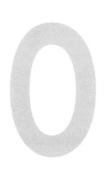

__pper

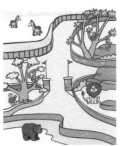

_ig_ag

27. The Sound Garden

Say the names of the animals in the garden. Listen for the first sound in each word. Then draw a line from each animal to the matching letter.

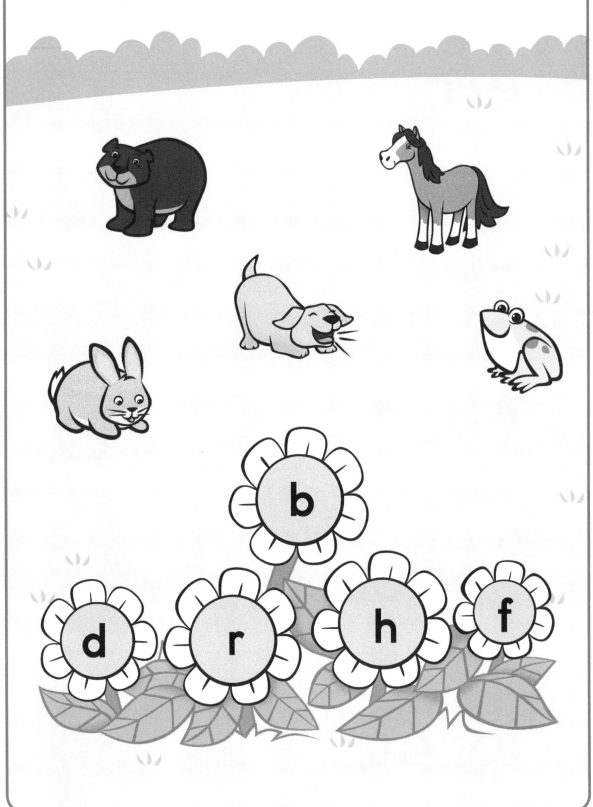

28. Galloping Greg

Help Greg the horse find everything in the picture that starts with the **g** sound. Circle each one you find!

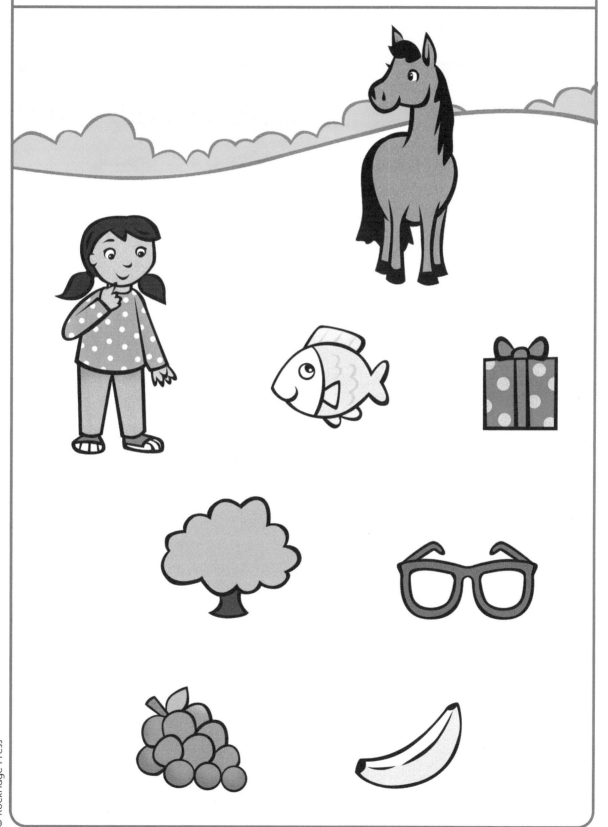

29. What's in the Fishbowl?

Color the objects in the bowl that begin with the **f** sound.

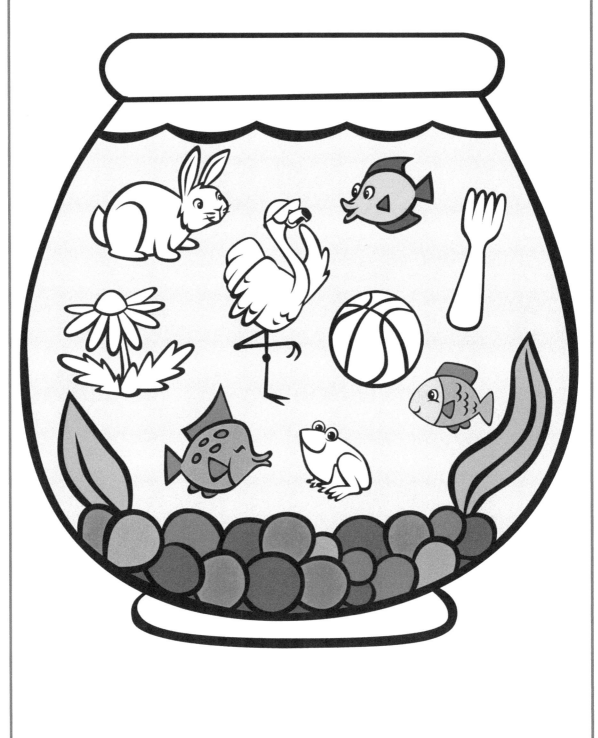

My Kindergarten Reading Workbook

30. Missing Letters

Write the letter for each missing beginning sound.

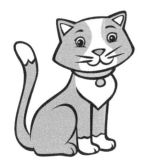 _____ at

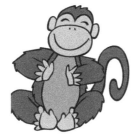 _____ onkey

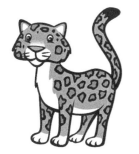 _____ aguar

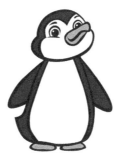 _____ enguin

 _____ amp

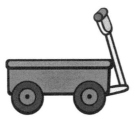 _____ agon

31. Swim in the Sea

Help the kids get to the sea! Follow the objects that start with the **s** sound.

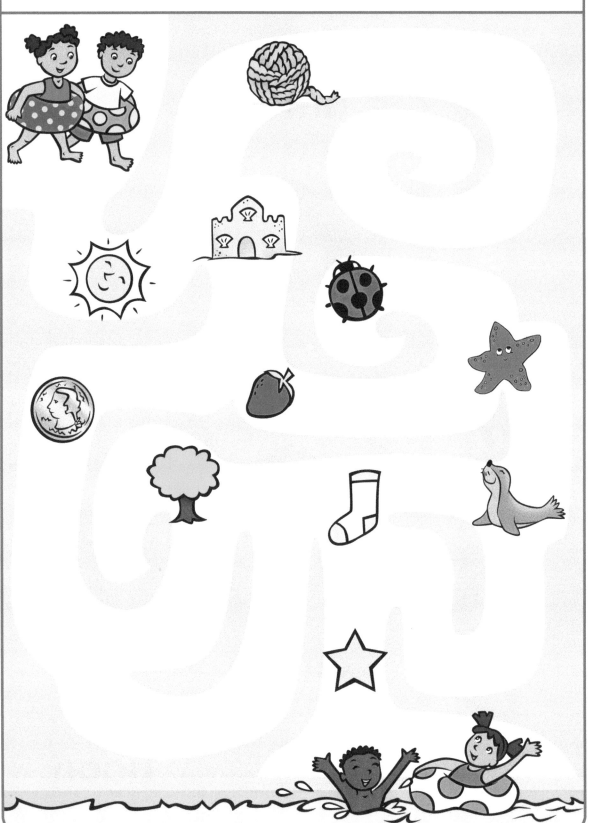

My Kindergarten Reading Workbook

32. Bone Hunt

Say the word for the picture on top of each bone. Listen for the end sound in the word. Then use the key to color each bone.

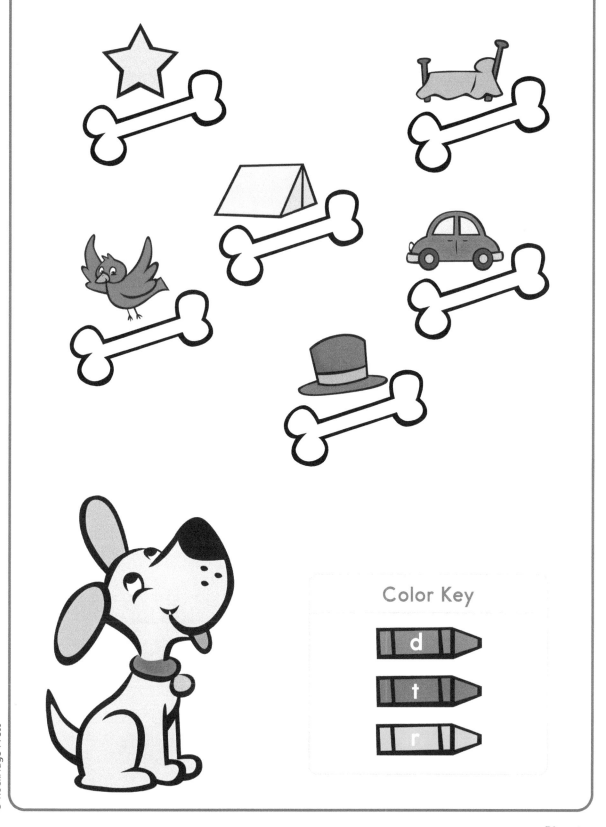

Color Key

d

t

r

33. Match the Ends

Say the name of each picture. Listen for the end sound in the word. Then draw a line from the picture to the sound.

b

n

p

m

l

r

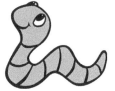

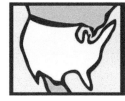

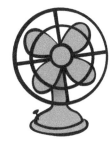

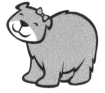

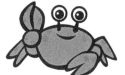

34. Brett in the Boat

Help Brett Bear fish for objects. Circle each one that ends with the **t** sound!

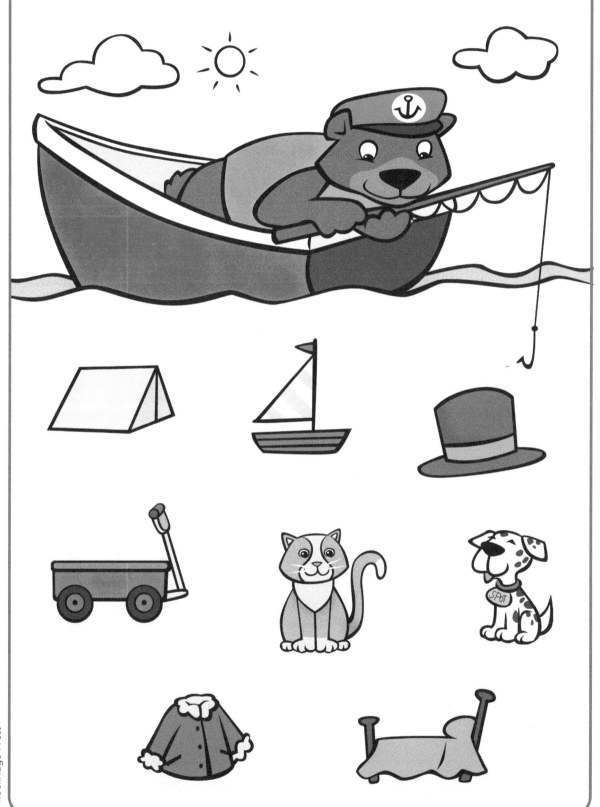

35. Listen for X!

Which objects end with the letter **X**? Find and color each one to get **3** in a row!

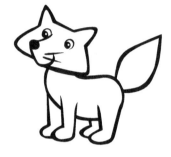 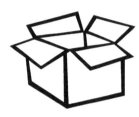 

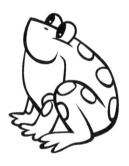 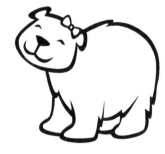 

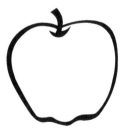 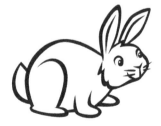 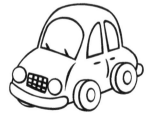

My Kindergarten Reading Workbook

36. What Is Missing?

The sounds are missing from the ends of the words! Write the letter of each missing sound.

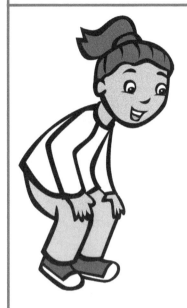

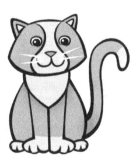

tu _____

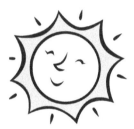

su _____

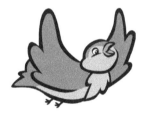

bir _____

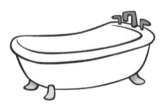

ca _____

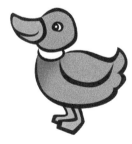

duc _____

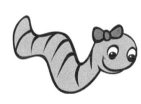

wor _____

37. Choo Choo!

Say each word in the puzzle. Do you hear the short **a** sound? Or do you hear the long **a** sound? Listen and then use the guide to color the picture.

Long a   Short a

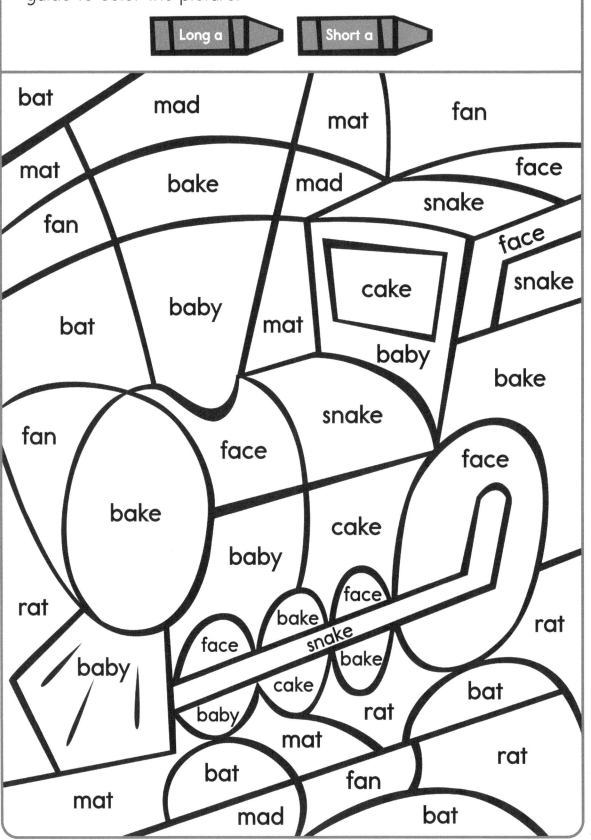

My Kindergarten Reading Workbook

38. Lost in Space

Help Andy Astronaut find the long and short **a** words in the puzzle.

l	a	r	m	e	r	f	r
l	c	a	t	u	f	h	a
i	q	i	k	p	c	o	g
h	u	n	d	e	r	u	n
g	h	a	t	d	h	s	o
a	k	r	l	y	k	e	r
m	n	l	p	e	o	k	n
e	m	r	a	k	e	l	a

Word Bank

cat
hat
rake
game
rain

39. Listen for the Long Sound!

Color the pictures that have a long **e** sound. Three in a row makes tic-tac-toe!

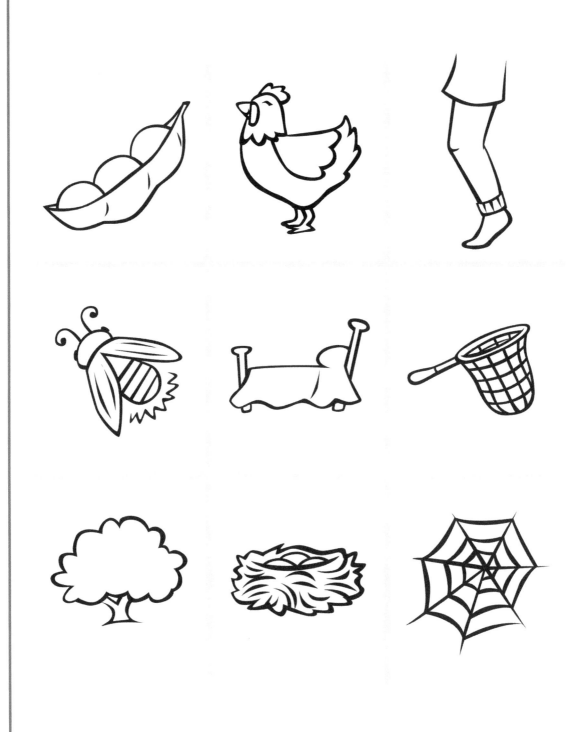

My Kindergarten Reading Workbook

40. Web of Words

Can you finish the crossword? Use the picture clues to help you fill in the puzzle. The words contain the long and short **e** sounds.

Word Bank

tent   tree
red   nest
pen

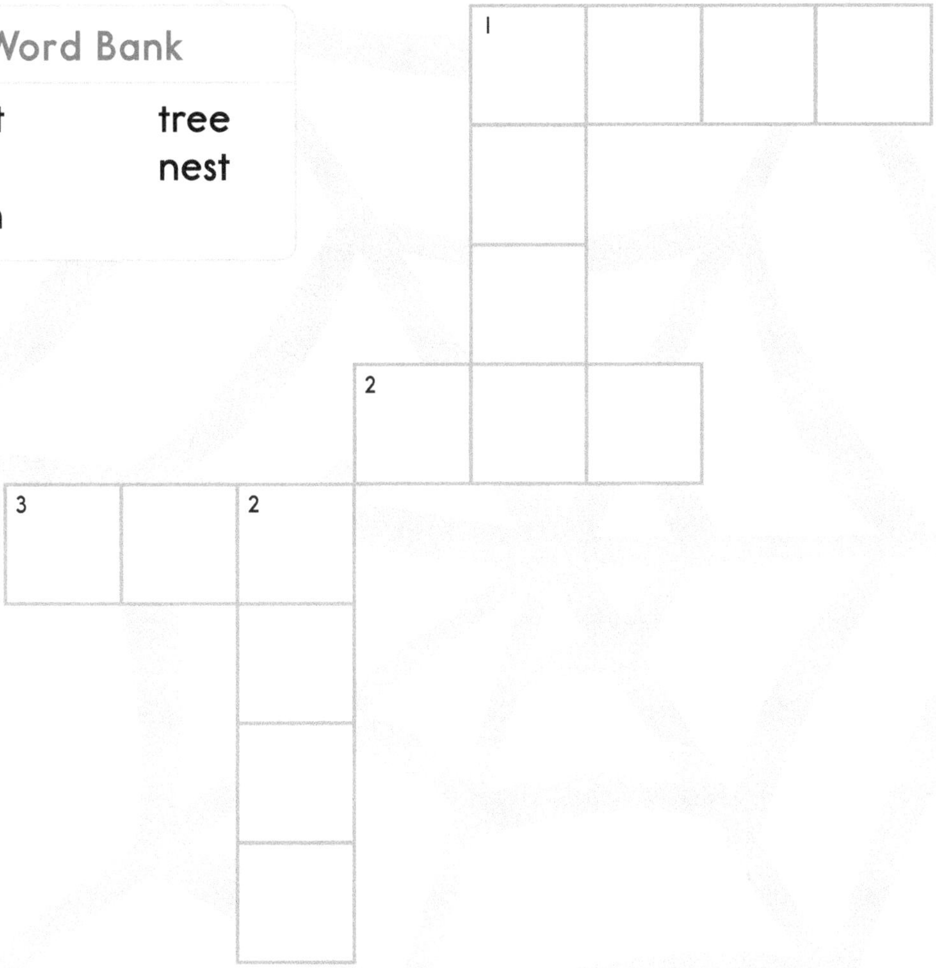

Across

1 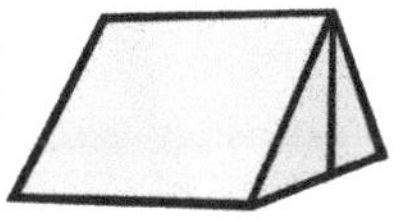   2 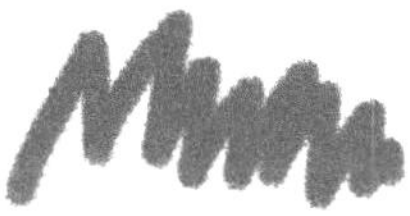   3

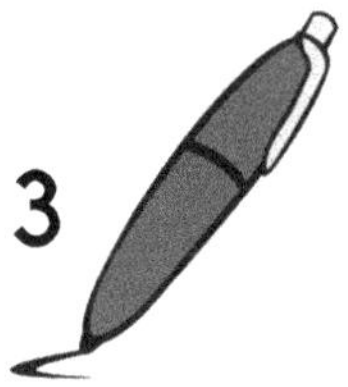

Down

1 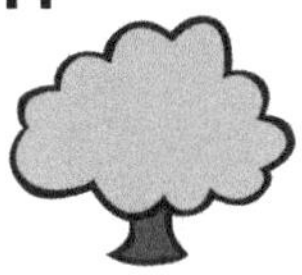   2

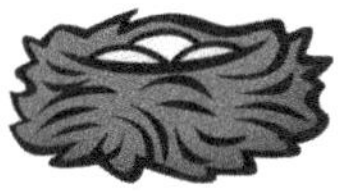

41. Short Surprise

Start at the star and draw a line to connect the dots. Say the word at each dot. Can you hear the short **i** sound? Color the picture when you are finished.

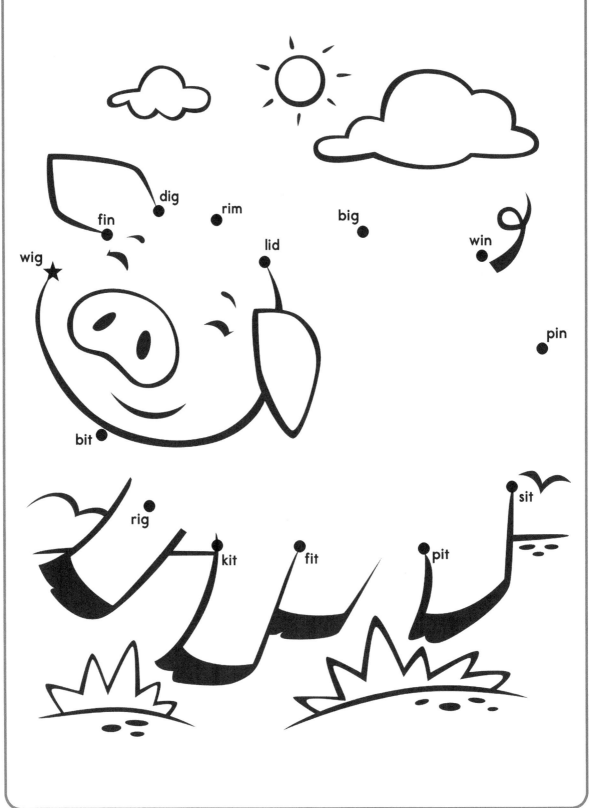

My Kindergarten Reading Workbook

42. Ice Cream Shop

Circle the ice cream cones with words that have the long i sound.

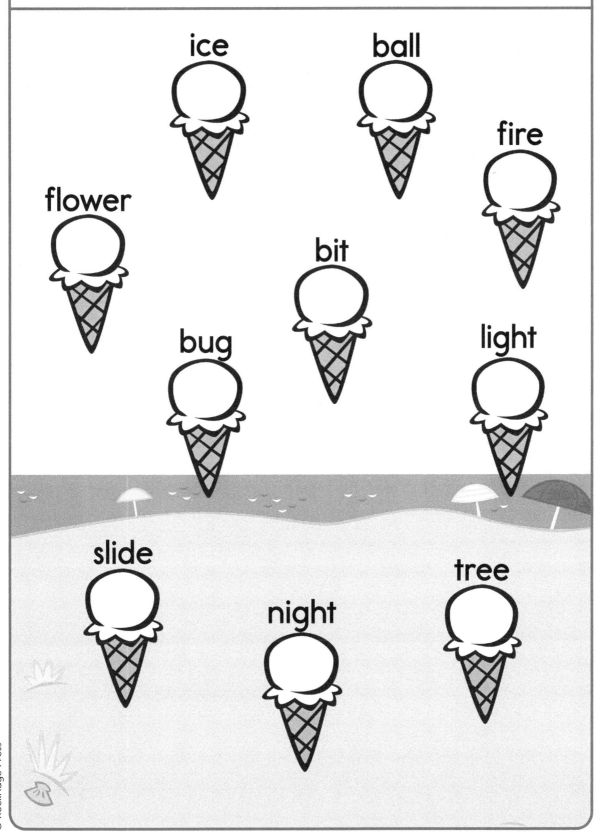

ice

ball

fire

flower

bit

bug

light

slide

night

tree

43. Climb Up the Tree

Help Otto get to his tree house! Follow the words with a short **o** sound to get through the maze.

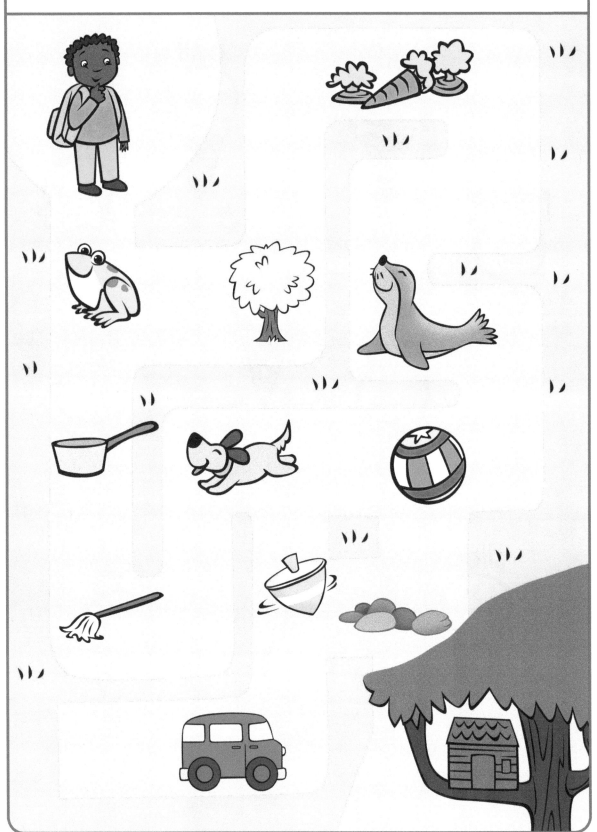

My Kindergarten Reading Workbook

© Rockridge Press

44. Snow Search

Use the picture clues to fill in the crossword puzzle. Each word has the long **o** sound.

Word Bank

cone
rope
rose
hose
boat

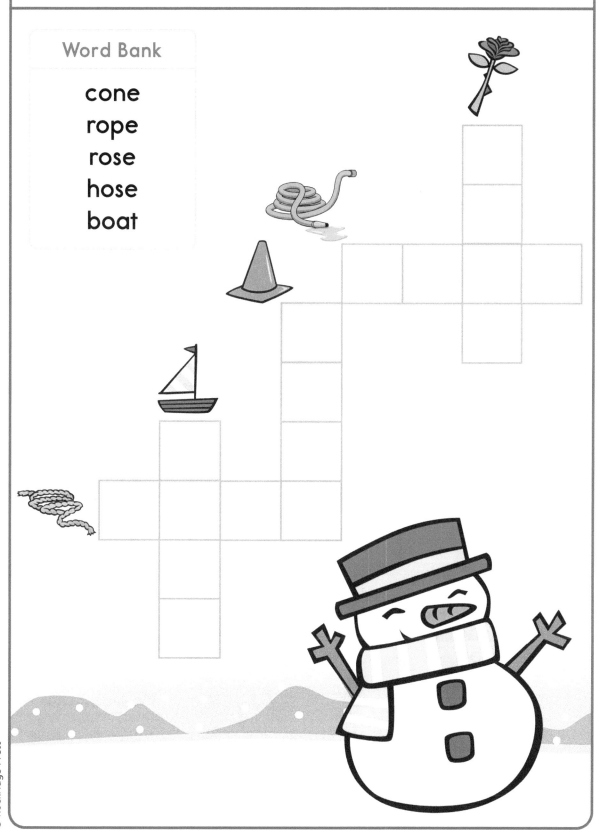

45. Unicorn Puzzle

Find and circle each word with a long **u** sound.

j	a	r	m	c	u	b	e
u	c	a	t	u	f	h	a
i	t	i	k	p	l	o	i
c	u	n	d	e	u	u	n
e	b	a	t	d	t	s	o
a	e	r	l	y	e	e	r
m	n	l	p	e	o	k	n
e	g	l	u	e	v	l	a

Word Bank

cube
glue
tube
flute
juice

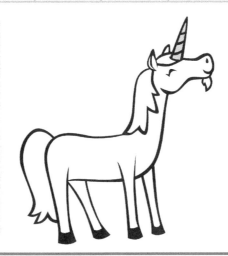

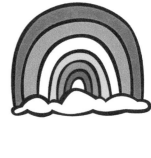

46. Bright Sun

Start at the star and connect the dots to finish the picture! Read the word at each dot. Do you hear the short **u** sound? Color the picture when you are finished.

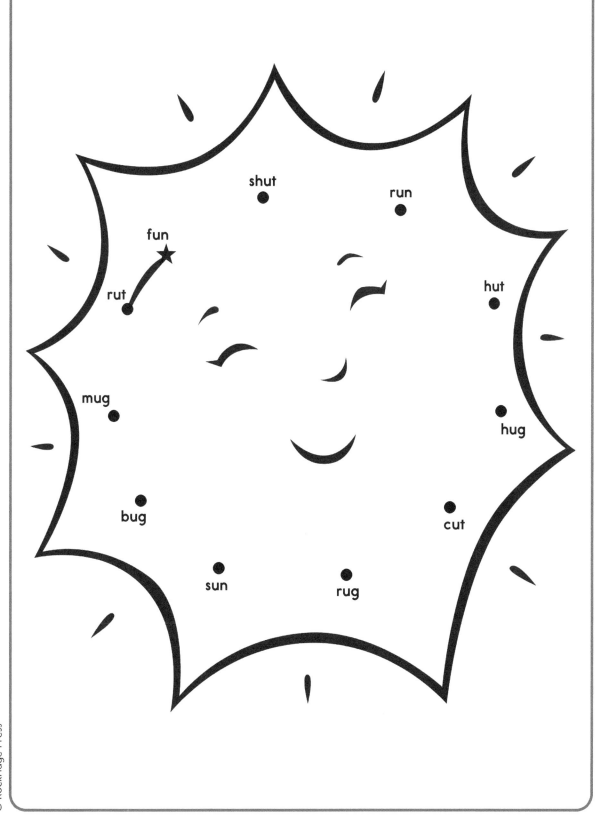

47. Bowl of Blends

Use the blends in the mixing bowl to complete each word.

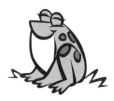

_____ **og**

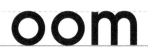

_____ **oom**

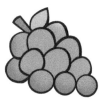

_____ **apes**

_____ **um**

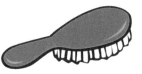

_____ **ush**

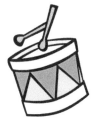

_____ **ass**

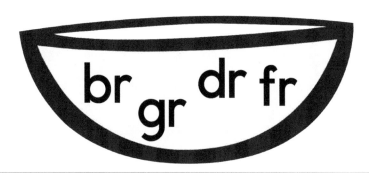

br gr dr fr

© Rockridge Press

48. Sliding In with L Blends

Fill in the missing letters of each word with an **l** blend to complete the puzzle. Use the pictures and blend bank to help you out.

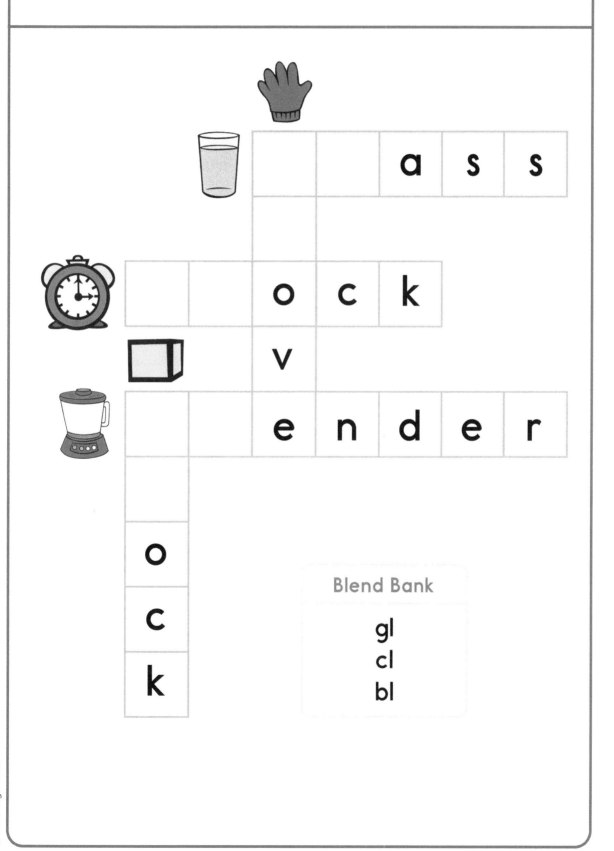

Blend Bank

gl
cl
bl

49. Shooting Stars

Circle the stars with pictures that begin with the **st** sound.

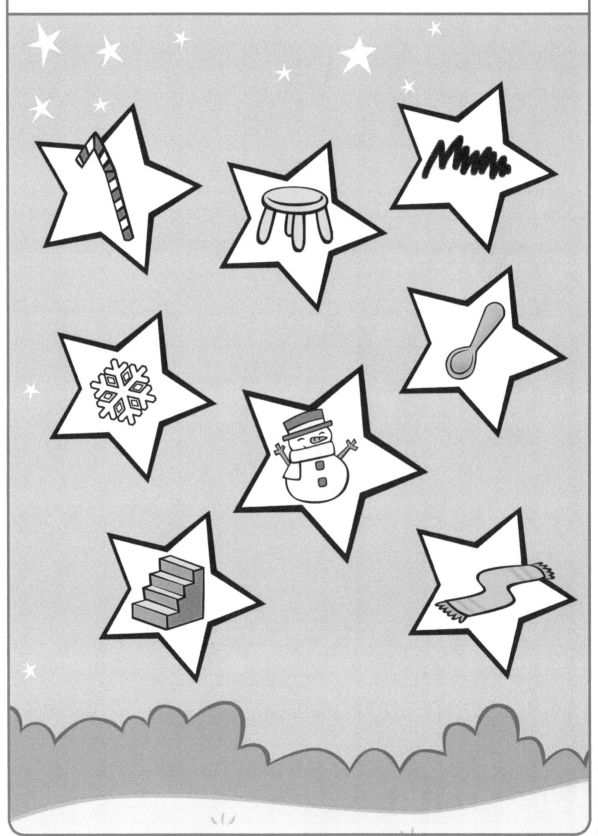

My Kindergarten Reading Workbook

50. Shark Search

Help Shelly Shark find each **sh** word hidden in the puzzle.

j	a	s	h	a	r	k	t
u	c	h	t	s	f	h	a
s	t	o	k	h	l	o	i
h	u	e	d	e	u	u	n
e	b	a	t	d	t	s	o
e	e	r	l	y	e	e	r
p	n	s	h	i	p	k	n
e	g	l	u	e	v	l	a

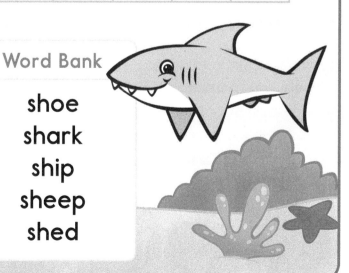

Word Bank

shoe
shark
ship
sheep
shed

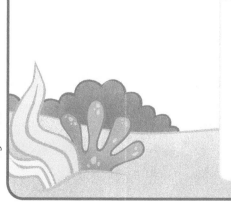

51. Henry Has a Hat

Start at the star and connect the dots to make a hat. Say the word at each dot and listen to the rhyme. Color the picture when you are finished.

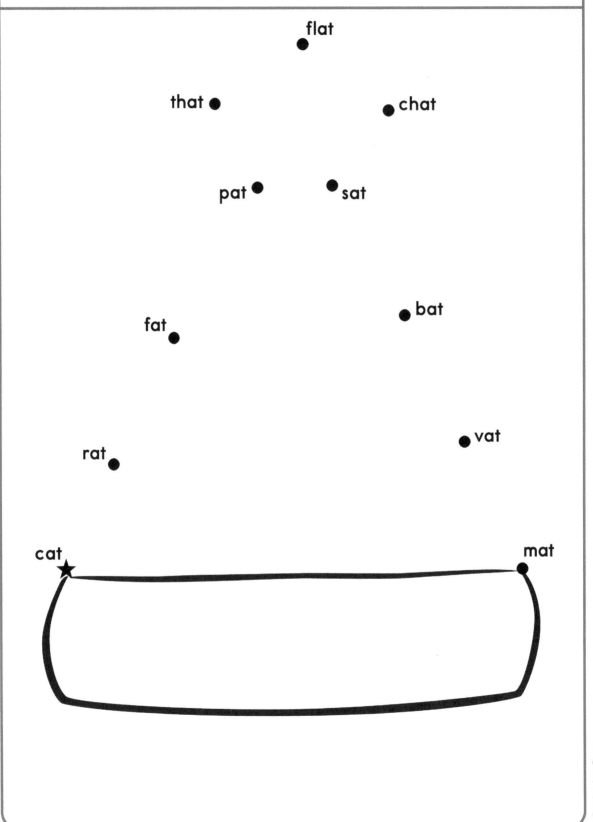

52. Room of Rhymes

Say the word on each crayon. Then use the guide to color the items that rhyme with each word.

What Rhymes with . . . ?

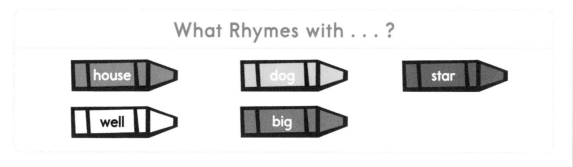

house | dog | star

well | big

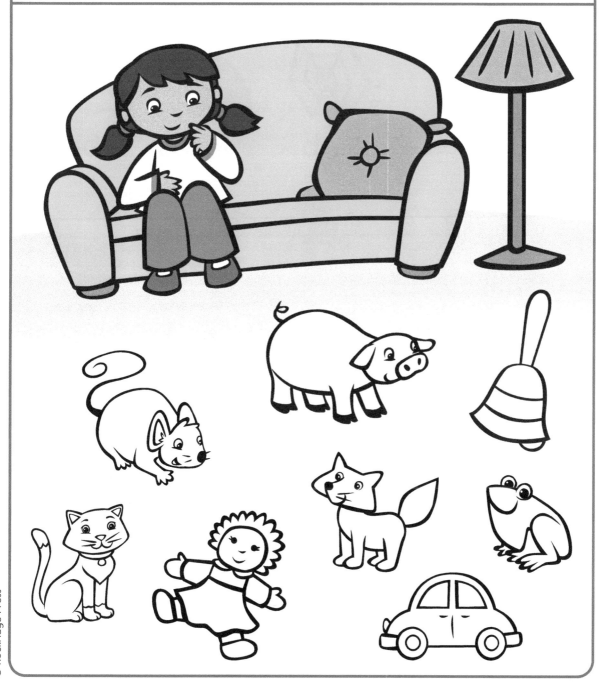

53. Scrambled Sounds

Unscramble the words. Then circle the object that rhymes in each row.

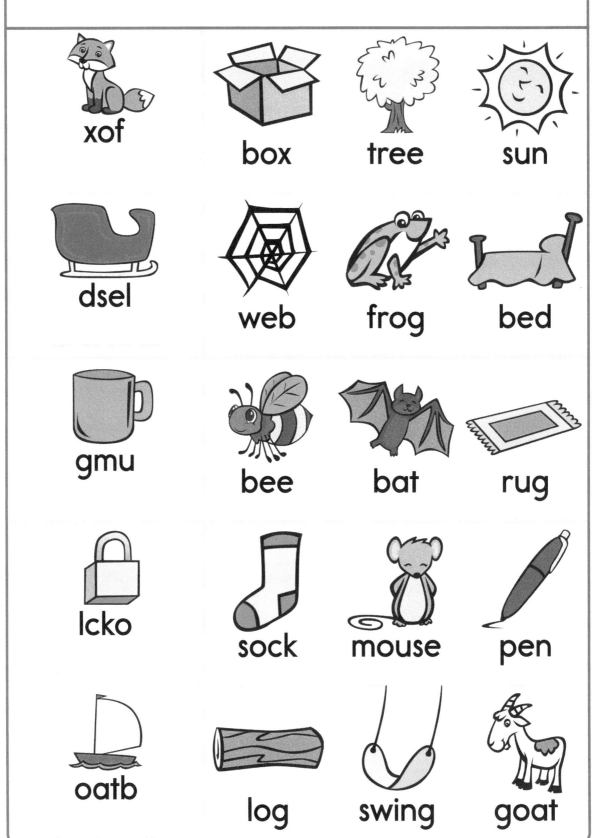

xof

box   tree   sun

dsel

web   frog   bed

gmu

bee   bat   rug

lcko

sock   mouse   pen

oatb

log   swing   goat

54. Race to the Finish!

Follow the objects that rhyme with **bug** to get through the maze.

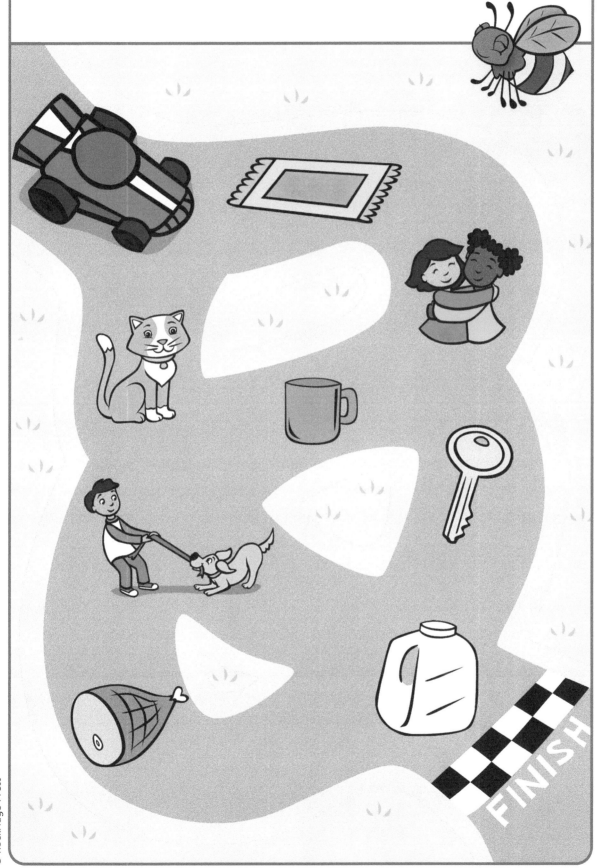

55. Score a Goal

Say the words on top of the soccer balls. Count the syllables in each word. Then draw a line from each word to the net with the matching number.

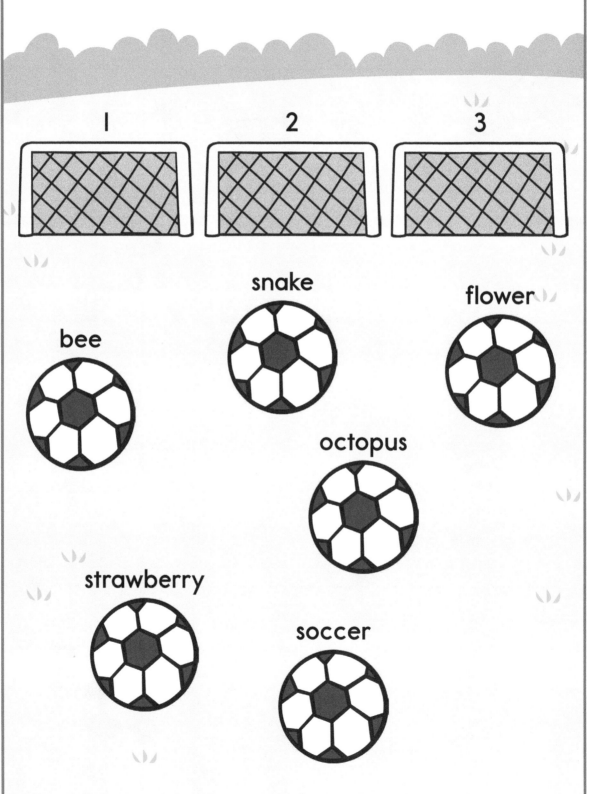

1   2   3

snake

bee

flower

octopus

strawberry

soccer

My Kindergarten Reading Workbook

© Rockridge Press

56. Dino Stomp

Help Daisy Dinosaur find and circle each object that has **2** syllables!

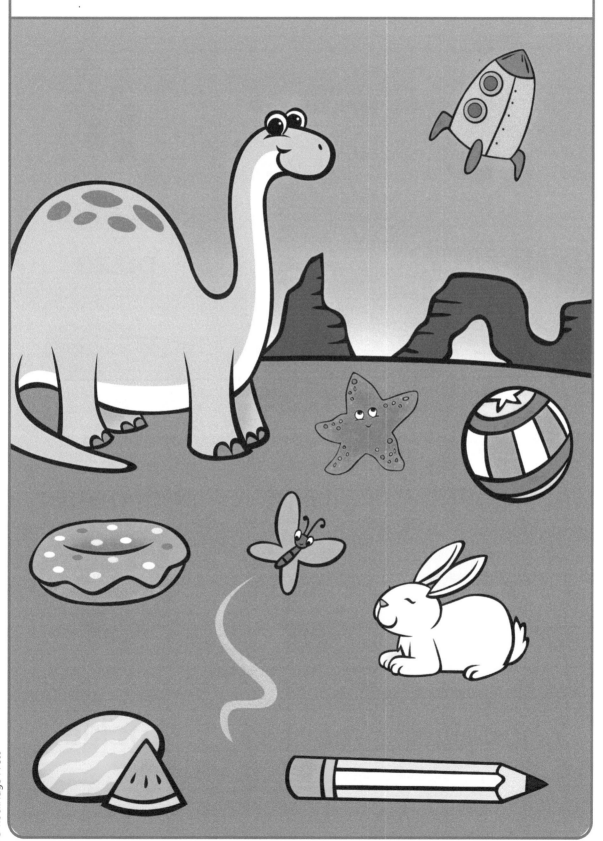

57. Sweet Snacks

Count the syllables in each word. Then color the cupcake with the correct number.

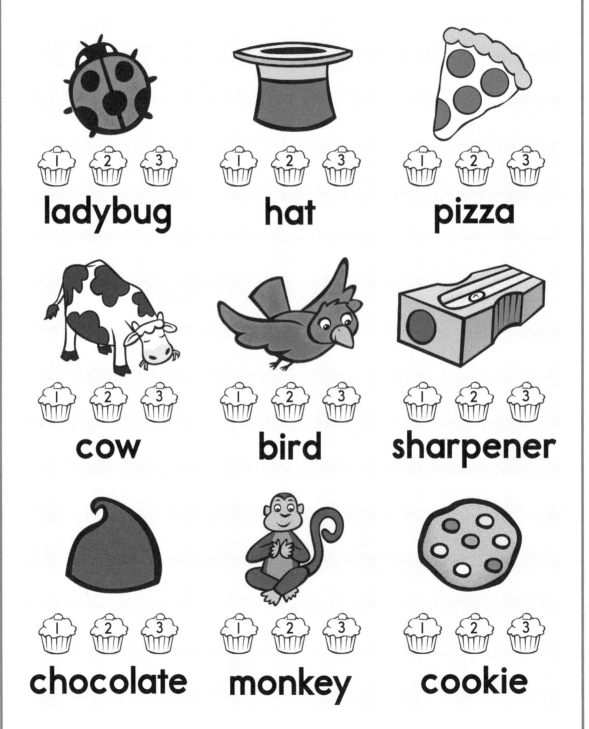

ladybug

hat

pizza

cow

bird

sharpener

chocolate

monkey

cookie

My Kindergarten Reading Workbook

© Rockridge Press

58. Single Syllable

Look at the pictures on the tic-tac-toe board. Color each picture that has **1** syllable.

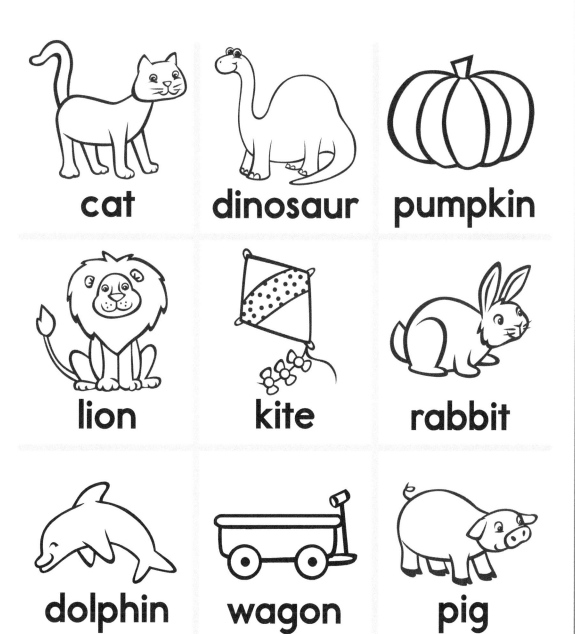

cat	dinosaur	pumpkin
lion	kite	rabbit
dolphin	wagon	pig

59. On the Farm

The farm is filled with sight words! Say each word on the page. Then use the guide to color the picture.

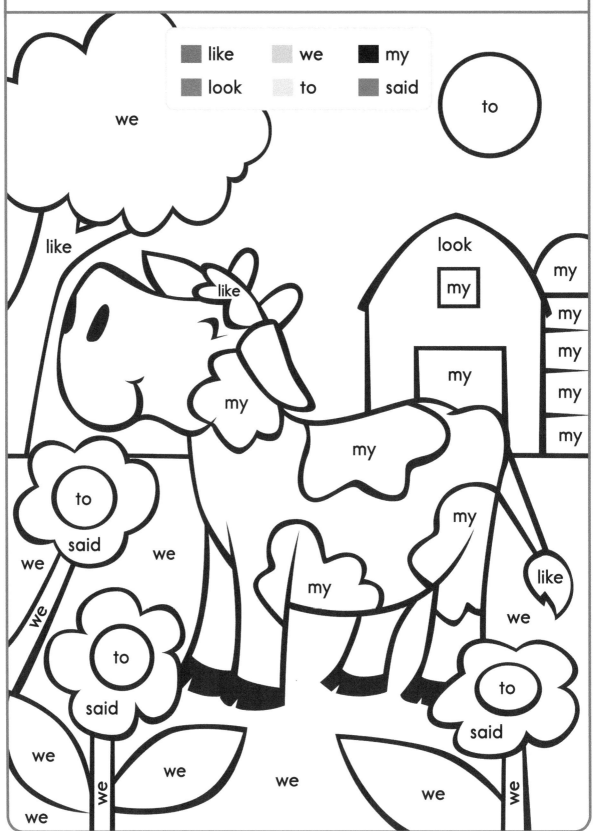

like	we	my
look	to	said

68   My Kindergarten Reading Workbook

60. Honeybee Hive

Start at the star and follow the word **have** to connect the dots. Color the picture when you finish!

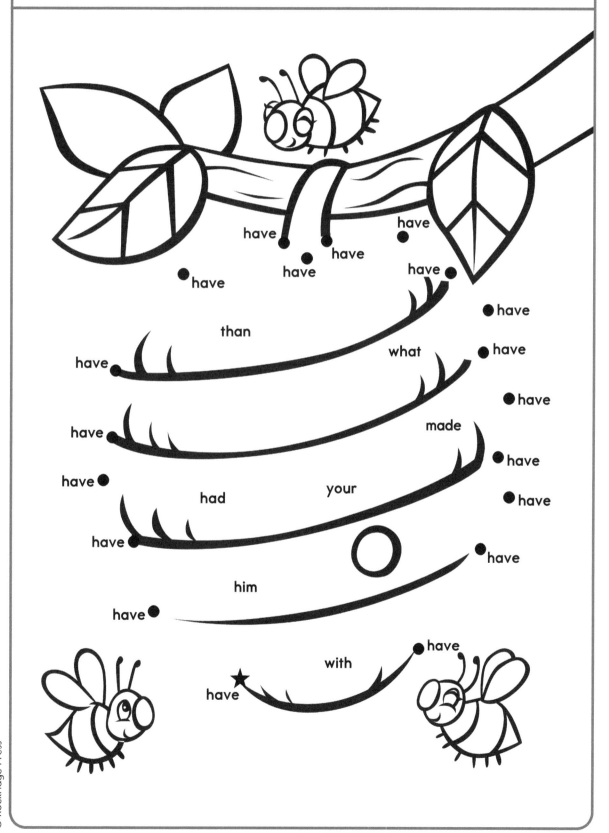

61. Take a Look!

The word **look** is hidden **5** times in the puzzle. Find and circle each word. Color a star after you find each word.

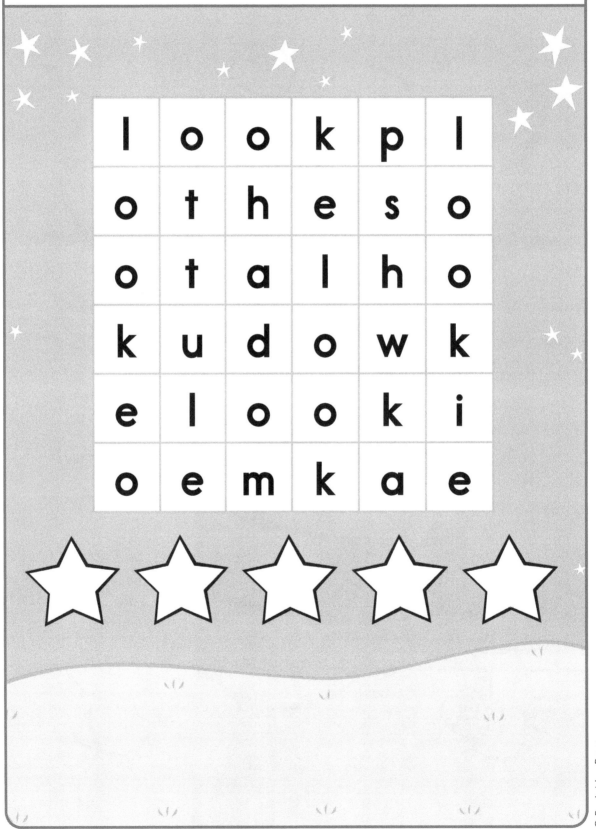

62. What Do You See?

Follow the words **see** and **it** to help Mama Bear reach her cave.

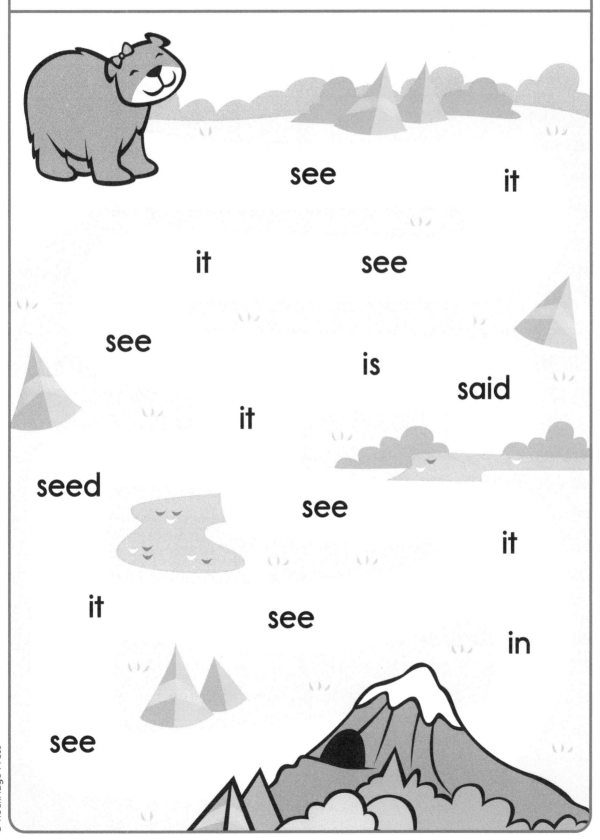

see

it

it

see

see

is

said

it

seed

see

it

it

see

in

see

63. Come and Swim!

Read the sight words in this picture. Then circle each word using the color key.

Color Key

■ what ■ come

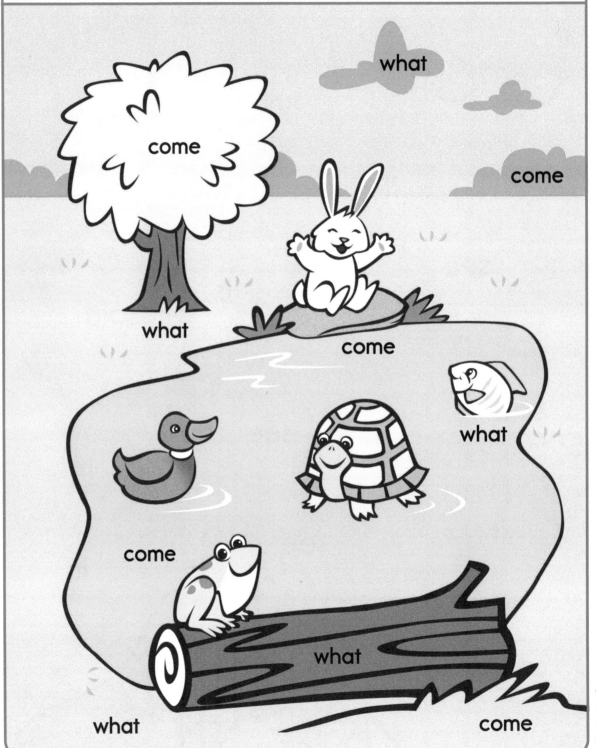

64. Burger and Fries

Draw a line to connect each burger to the matching fries. Color the pictures when you are finished!

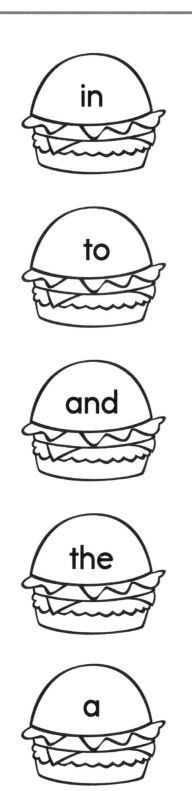

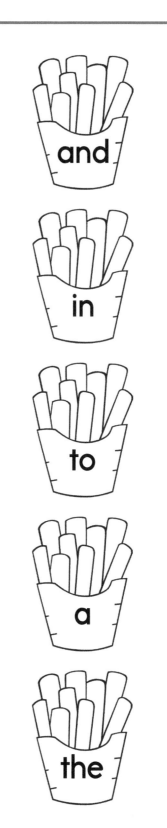

65. Crossword Fun

Use the word bank to finish each sentence and fill in the puzzle.

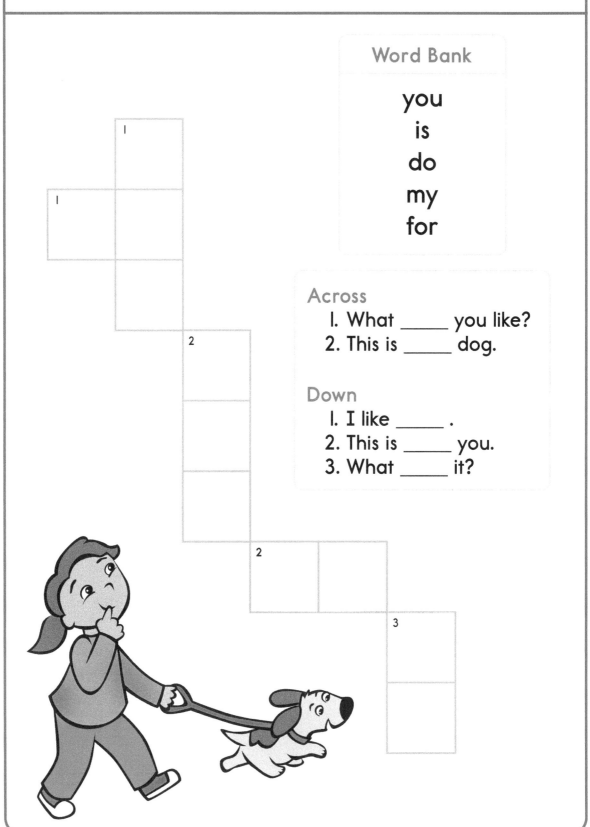

Word Bank

you

is

do

my

for

Across
1. What _____ you like?
2. This is _____ dog.

Down
1. I like _____ .
2. This is _____ you.
3. What _____ it?

66. Three in a Row

Find the sight words that appear **3** times in each tic-tac-toe board. Then draw a line through them to make a row!

that	for	have	is	be	in
my	that	a	my	be	that
we	see	that	to	be	that

be	for	was	are	can	to
my	was	see	are	a	have
was	as	it	are	that	that

in	for	as	is	with	we
my	that	as	me	with	like
we	see	as	to	with	like

67. In the Grass

Read the sight words. Then find and circle each word in the puzzle.

j	a	s	h	p	l	l	t
u	c	a	t	s	f	o	a
t	t	i	k	h	l	o	i
p	u	d	o	w	u	k	n
g	b	a	u	d	t	s	o
o	e	m	t	y	e	e	r
p	n	e	h	i	p	k	n
e	g	l	u	e	a	l	l

Word Bank

said   look   all
me   go   out

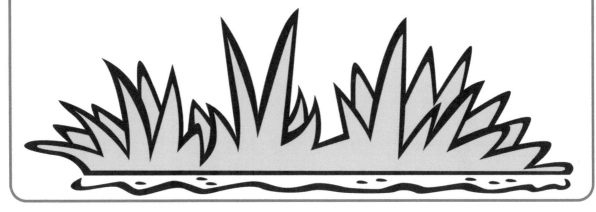

My Kindergarten Reading Workbook

68. Sight Word Scramble!

Use the word bank to unscramble and write each word.

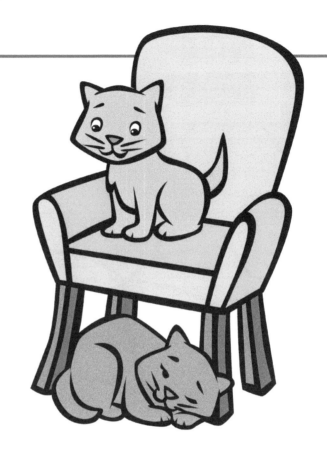

Word Bank

they
at
this
one
had
from

stih	rfom	tyeh

noe	ta	dah

69. In the Ocean

Color the fish using the color key.

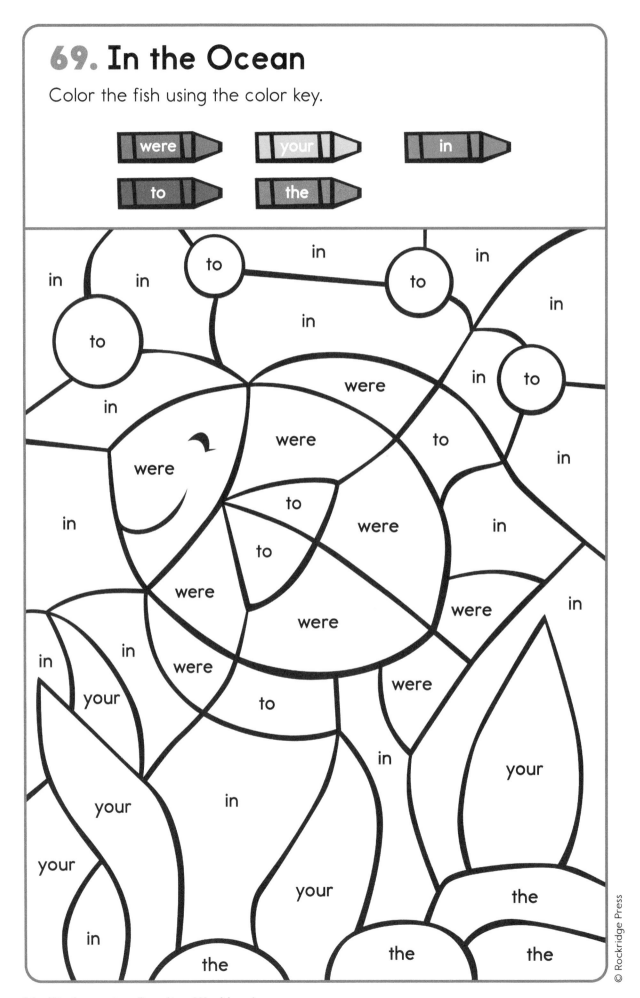

My Kindergarten Reading Workbook

© Rockridge Press

70. Down the Hill

Can you find the sight words in this puzzle? Be sure to look across and down.

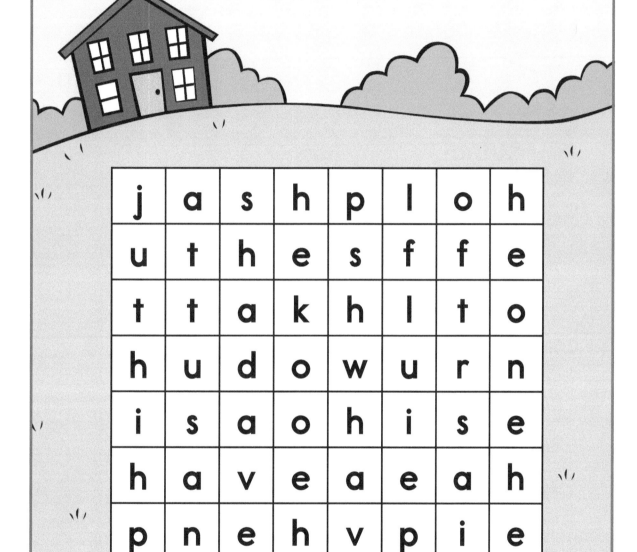

j	a	s	h	p	l	o	h
u	t	h	e	s	f	f	e
t	t	a	k	h	l	t	o
h	u	d	o	w	u	r	n
i	s	a	o	h	i	s	e
h	a	v	e	a	e	a	h
p	n	e	h	v	p	i	e
e	d	o	w	n	a	d	r

Word Bank

down   the   have
one   had

71. I Can Fly!

Help the bird fly back to her nest! Follow and trace the word **can** to get through the maze.

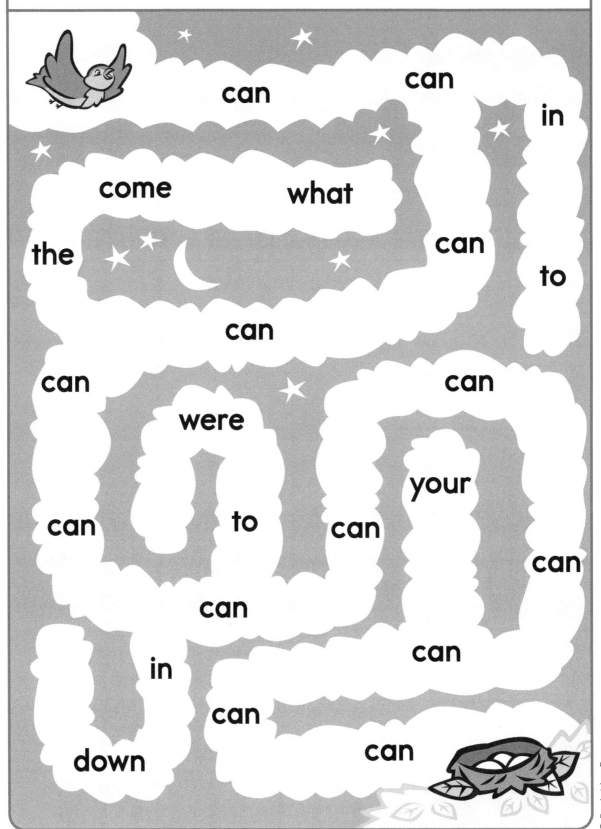

My Kindergarten Reading Workbook

© Rockridge Press

72. Crunchy Apples

Read the sight word on each apple. Find the basket with the matching word. Draw a line to connect each apple with the correct basket.

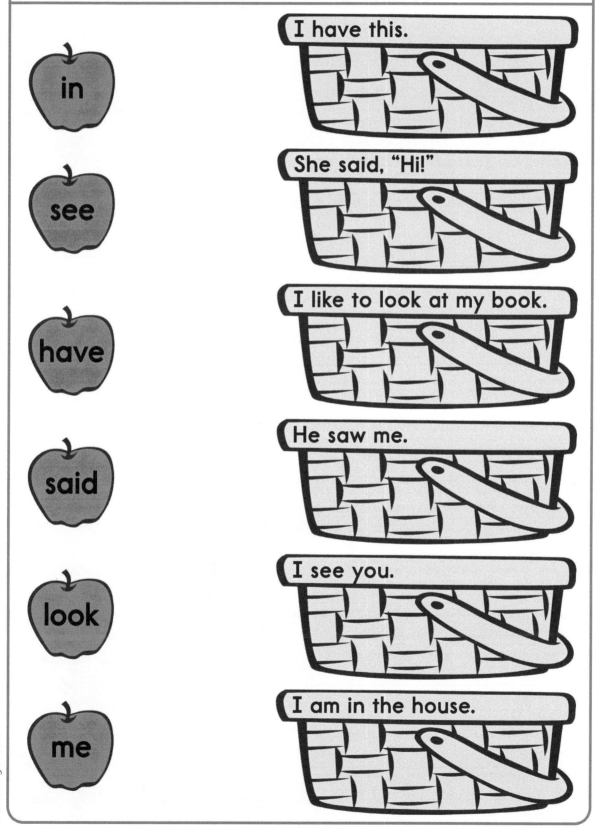

in

see

have

said

look

me

I have this.

She said, "Hi!"

I like to look at my book.

He saw me.

I see you.

I am in the house.

73. Read and Write Sight Words

Use the word bank to find the missing word in each sentence. Then write the correct words to finish the puzzle.

Across
1. Let's go _____ the store.
2. He is there. Can you get _____ a fork?

Down
1. Where is _____ pen?
2. She is nice. Here is _____ book.
3. I have this _____ that.

Word Bank

to

and

the

him

her

74. Time for Tic-Tac-Toe

Draw a line through the sight words that appear **3** times in each tic-tac-toe board. Three in a row wins!

my	for	for	is	go	in
my	that	a	do	do	do
my	see	can	to	see	see

all	all	all	out	to	to
my	my	see	out	a	have
down	as	it	out	that	come

in	for	like	is	can	we
my	like	as	me	can	like
like	see	as	to	can	like

75. The Wishing Well

Find and circle each sight word in the puzzle. Be sure to look across and down. Make a wish when you finish!

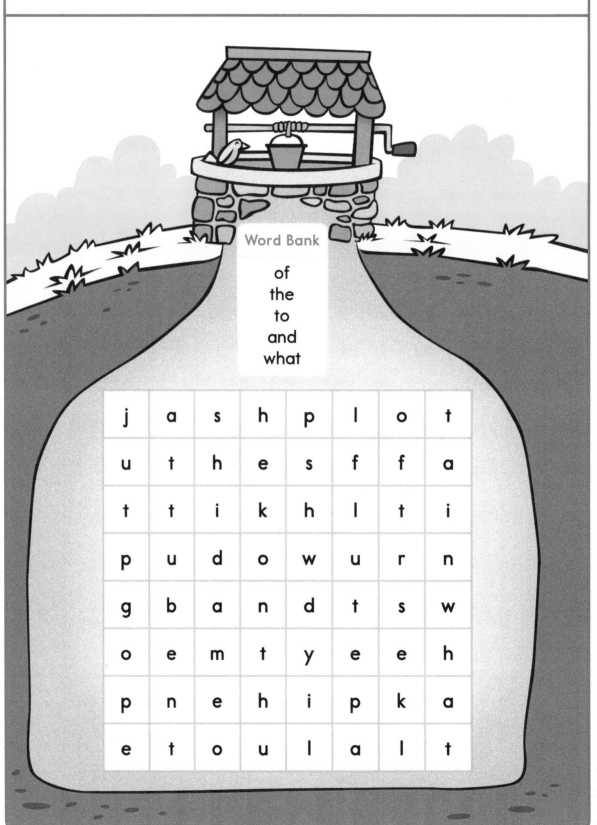

Word Bank

of
the
to
and
what

j	a	s	h	p	l	o	t
u	t	h	e	s	f	f	a
t	t	i	k	h	l	t	i
p	u	d	o	w	u	r	n
g	b	a	n	d	t	s	w
o	e	m	t	y	e	e	h
p	n	e	h	i	p	k	a
e	t	o	u	l	a	l	t

76. Jumbled Up

Unscramble and write each word. Use the word bank to help you.

reh ☐ ☐ ☐

shi ☐ ☐ ☐

ouy ☐ ☐ ☐

ew ☐ ☐

em ☐ ☐

ocme ☐ ☐ ☐ ☐

Word Bank

her   his   you   we   me   come

77. Fish Tank Fun

Color each fish in the tank using the color key.

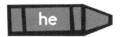 he   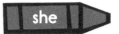 she

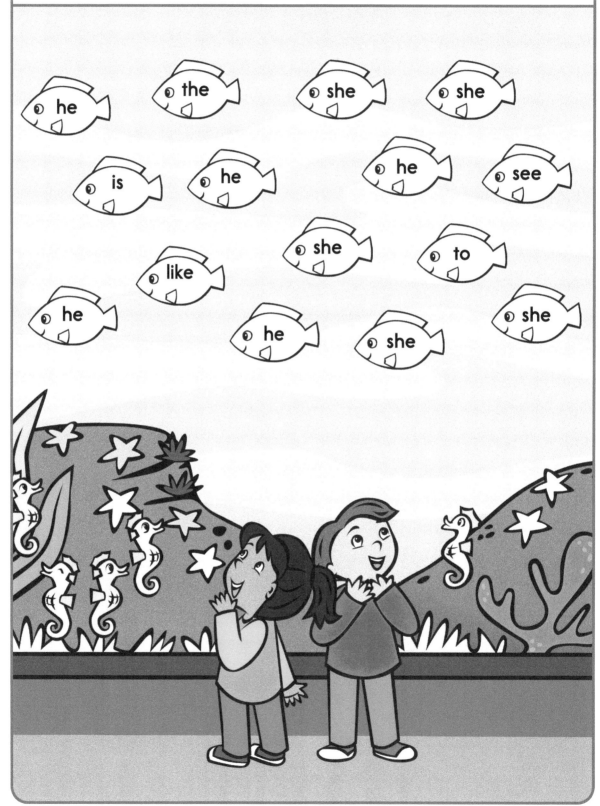

78. Strike Out Sight Words

Put an X over the sight words that appear **3** times in each tic-tac-toe board.

and	and	and
to	to	a
we	see	are

is	what	in
my	what	that
to	what	that

be	for	then
my	then	see
then	as	it

are	can	to
are	a	have
by	by	by

am	for	as
my	am	as
we	see	am

is	will	we
me	will	like
to	will	like

79. A Sunny Day

Start at the star. Connect the dots and say each sight word out loud to finish the sentence. What do you see when you connect the dots? Color the picture when you are finished.

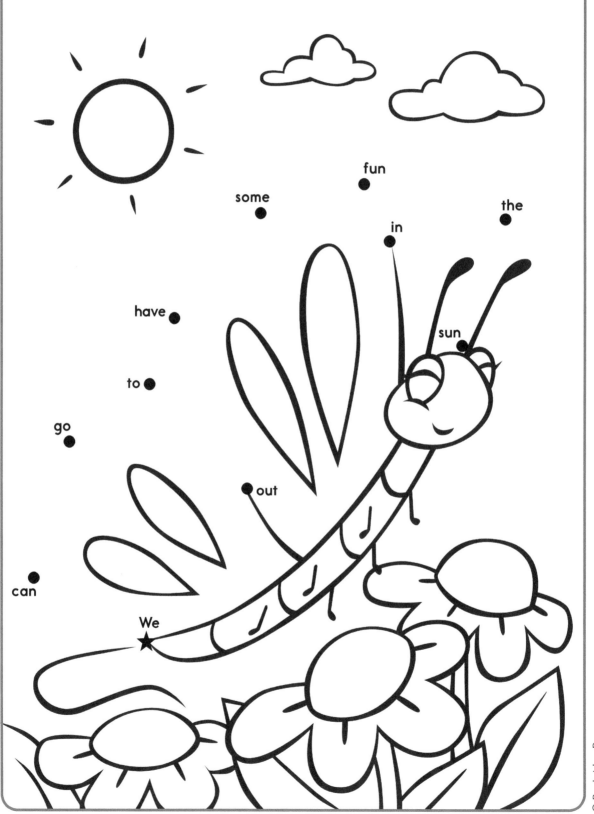

fun

some

in

the

have

sun

to

go

out

can

We

My Kindergarten Reading Workbook

© Rockridge Press

80. Milk and Cookies

Time for a snack! Start at the milk carton and color the boxes with the word **said** to get to the cookie. YUM!

	said	we	said	said	said
go	said	for	said	me	said
the	said	said	said	is	said
a	are	down	said	said	said
to	like	her	he	said	my
you	this	it	you	said	

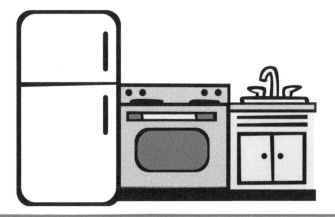

81. Up, Up, and Away

Read the words in the balloons. Then draw lines to connect the matching balloons. Color the pictures when you are finished.

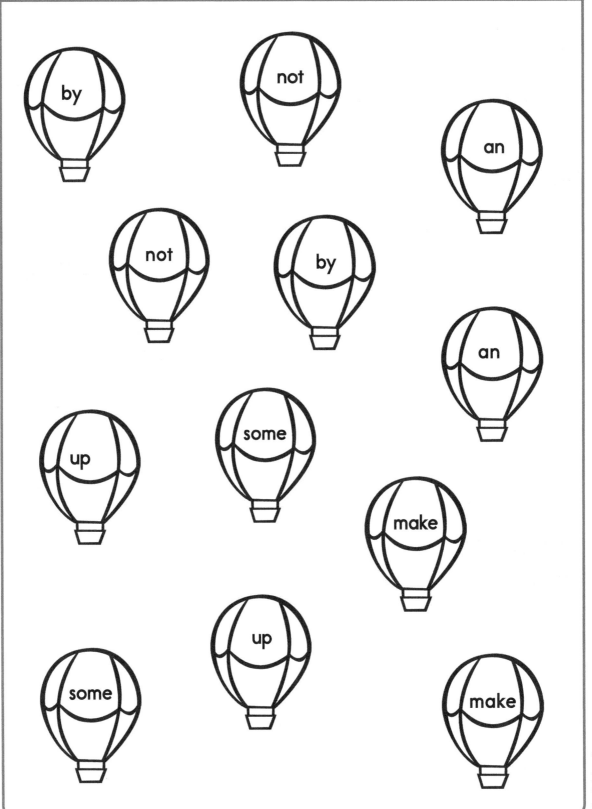

My Kindergarten Reading Workbook

82. Clown Around

Can you solve the crossword? Use the word bank to find the missing word in each sentence.

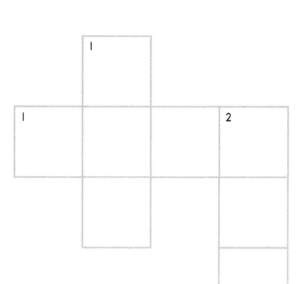

Across
1. The apple is _____ .
2. I _____ do it!

Down
1. _____ are you?
2. I fell _____ .
3. _____ is big.

Word Bank

how
good
this
down
can

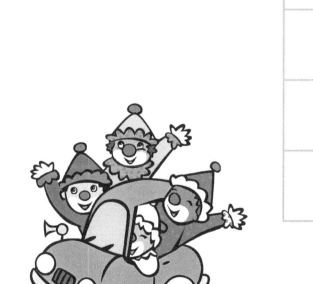

83. Castle Search

Find and circle each word in the puzzle!

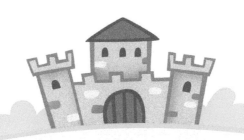

j	a	s	h	p	l	o	h
u	t	h	r	s	f	f	e
t	t	e	l	h	l	t	g
p	u	d	o	w	u	r	n
g	s	a	o	h	i	s	w
o	e	m	k	y	e	a	h
p	n	e	h	i	p	i	e
e	t	o	u	l	a	d	r

Word Bank

he   she   her
his   look   said

84. Where Is the Bird?

Circle the words that match each picture.

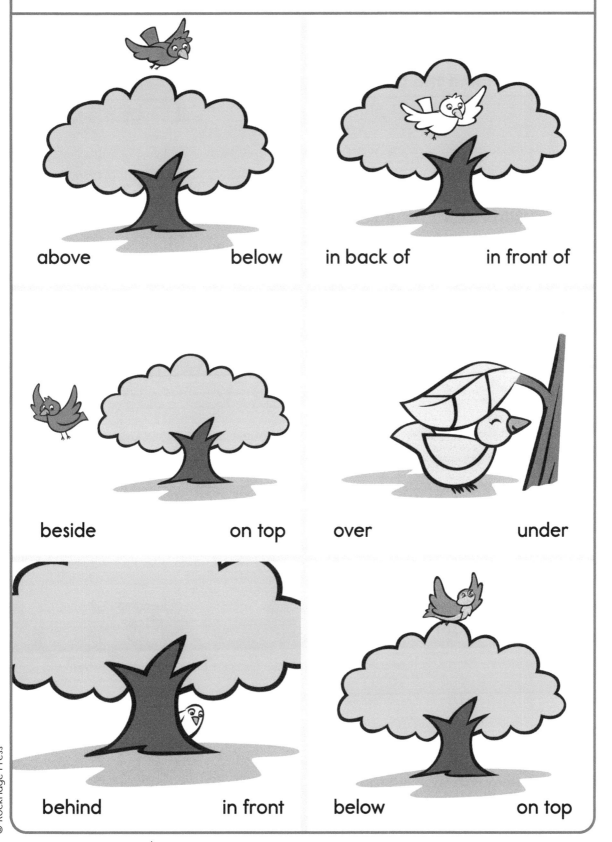

above   below   in back of   in front of

beside   on top   over   under

behind   in front   below   on top

© Rockridge Press

85. Leo Lion

Read the sentences below. Then draw a line to match each sentence to its picture.

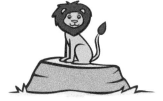

Leo is behind the grass.

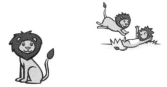

Leo is in front of the rock.

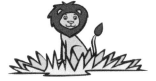

Leo is next to the water.

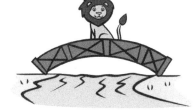

Leo is on top of the rock.

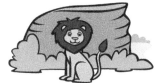

Leo is far from his friends.

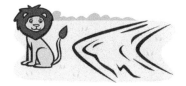

Leo is over the water.

86. Color the Pairs

Read the words on the page. Find and color each pair of opposite words. Use the same color for each opposite pair.

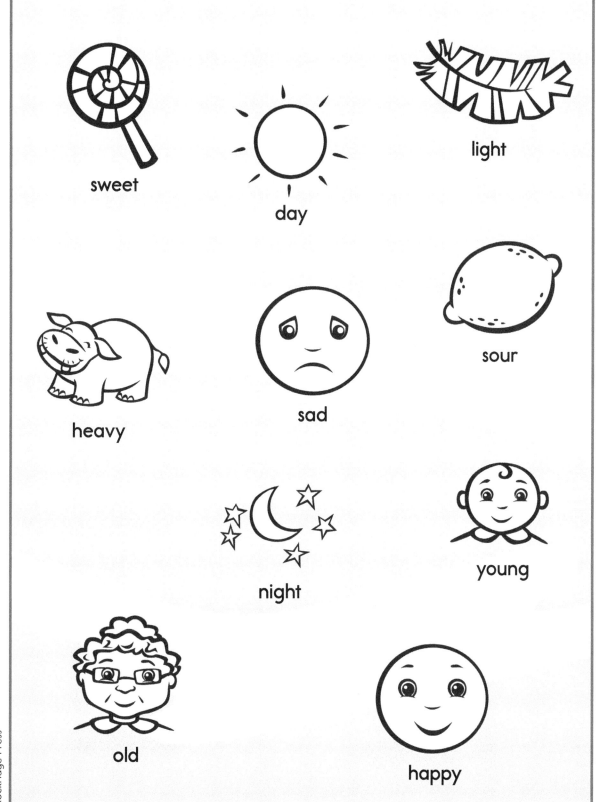

sweet

day

light

heavy

sad

sour

night

young

old

happy

87. Matching Opposites

Read each word in the left column. Then draw a line to the opposite word in the right column.

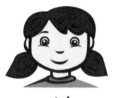

girl

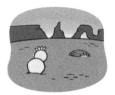

dry

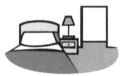

full

boy

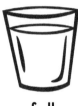

bright

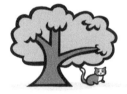

down

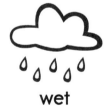

wet

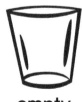

empty

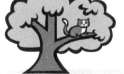

up

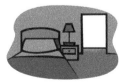

dark

My Kindergarten Reading Workbook

88. Scrambled-Up Opposites

Read each word on the left. Then unscramble and write the word in each opposite pair.

little

gib

stand

tis

short

allt

cold

tho

slow

staf

Word Bank

hot   tall   fast   big   sit

89. A Day at the Park

Read each action word. Then find and circle the matching part of the picture.

Word Bank

hop
throw
read
eat
drive
paint

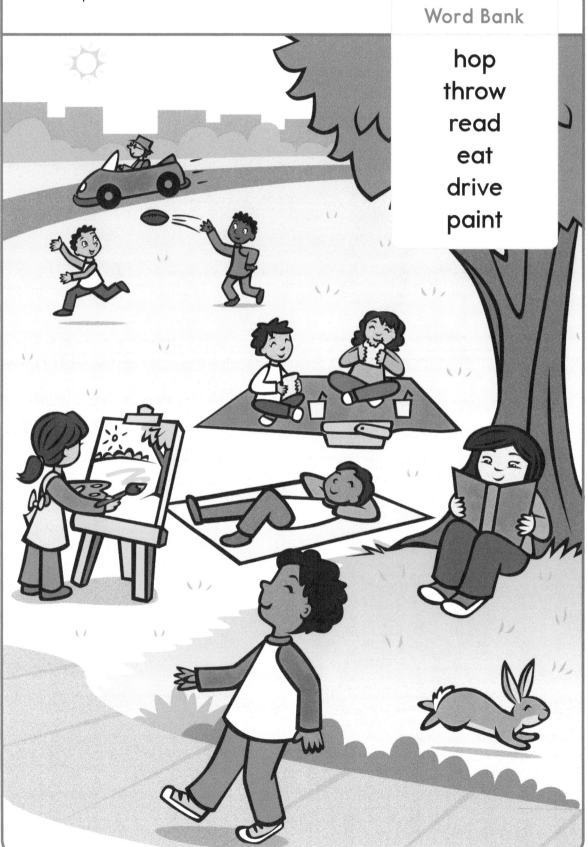

My Kindergarten Reading Workbook

90. Mixed-Up Words

Unscramble and write each action word. Use the word bank and pictures to help you.

Word Bank

jump   run   swim   climb   fly

nur _____   _____

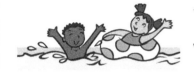

wmis _____   _____

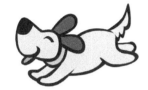

lfy _____   _____

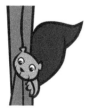

cmlib _____   _____

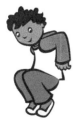

pumj _____   _____

91. Action Tic-Tac-Toe!

Read the sentences in each tic-tac-toe square. Put an X on each sentence that has an action word in it. Can you find **3** in a row?

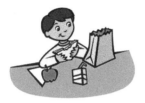
He eats lunch.

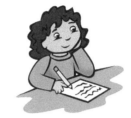
She writes poems.

He rides a bike.

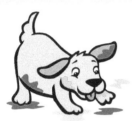
I like dogs.

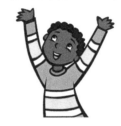
Where is he?

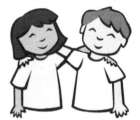
You are nice.

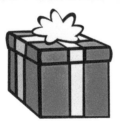
What is it?

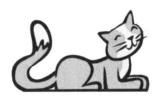
I have a cat.

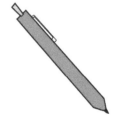
I like your pen.

92. The Dog

Read the story. Then circle the answer to each question below.

The Dog

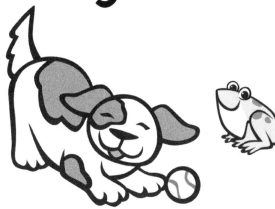

The dog is big.
The dog likes the frog.
The dog plays with a ball.

The dog is _____ .
Circle the answer in red.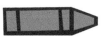
A. dog   B. cat   C. big

What does the dog like?
Circle the answer in green.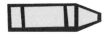
A. frog   B. bat   C. duck

What does the dog play with?
Circle the answer in yellow.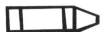
A. rock   B. ball   C. run

93. My Messy Desk

Read the sentences. Then color the picture to match each sentence.

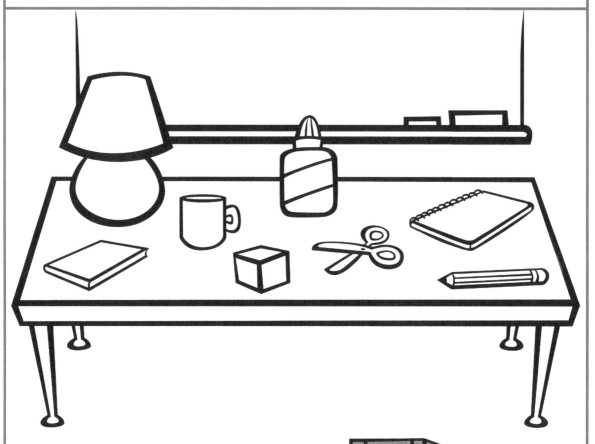

1. The mug is pink.

2. The glue is purple.

3. The lamp is gray.

4. The pencil is yellow.

5. The notebook is red.

6. The book is blue.

7. The box is brown.

8. The scissors are green.

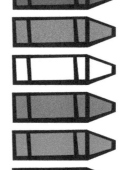

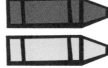

94. My Day

Read the story. Then unscramble and write the words from the story.

My Day

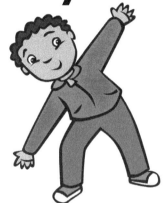

I go to school. I play
with Sam. I read books.
I go home. I eat pizza.

Word Bank

home
pizza
play
books
school

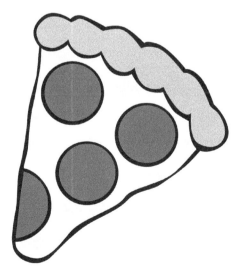

hoolsc

ylap

koosb

ohme

azzip

95. Fruit Bowl Fun!

Read the story. Then choose **3** questions in the tic-tac-toe board. Answer and circle **3** questions in a row to win!

My Fruit Bowl

Look at the basket! It is brown. I see a purple plum. The banana tastes good. Where is the apple? I see it! It is by the basket. I will eat the orange next.

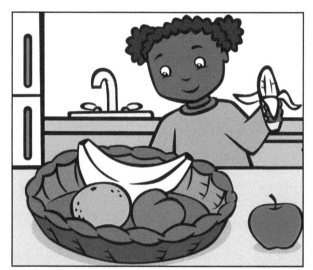

Where is the basket?	What color is the plum?	The banana tastes . . .
A. Floor	A. Green	A. Bad
B. Table	B. Pink	B. Okay
C. Sink	C. Purple	C. Good

Where is the apple?	What fruit will the girl eat next?	Where does the story take place?
A. Under the basket	A. Apple	A. Bathroom
B. Next to the basket	B. Orange	B. Kitchen
C. Over the basket	C. Grapes	C. Bedroom

Who eats the fruit?	What is the story about?	What color is the basket?
A. Mom	A. Fruit	A. Blue
B. Girl	B. Pizza	B. Brown
C. Boy	C. Vegetables	C. Black

© Rockridge Press

96. A Day at the Farm

Read the story. Then color the animals that were in the story.

A Day at the Farm

I am at the farm. I see many things. There is a cow.
There are pigs. Over there is a horse. I like the chickens.

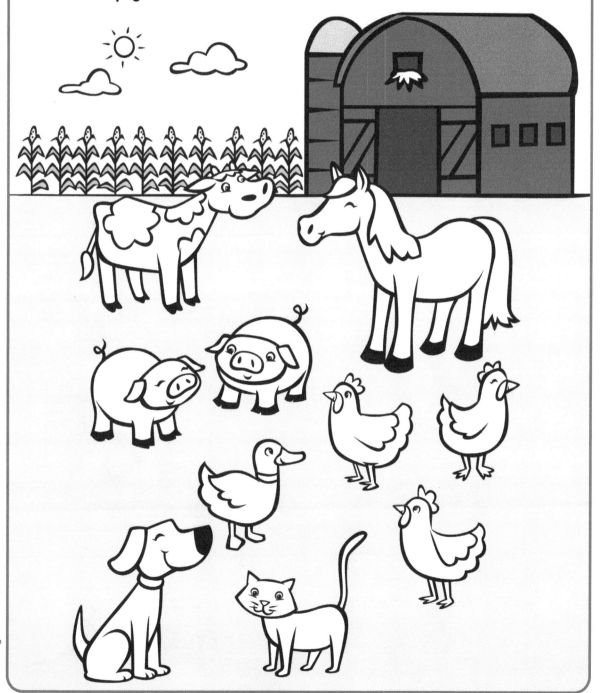

97. Read and Match

Draw a line from each sentence to the matching picture.

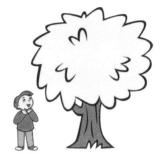

The bird can fly.

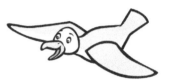

I see a frog on a log.

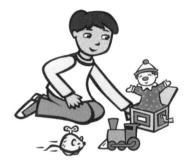

I like to read on my bed.

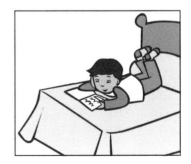

I like to play with my toys.

Look at that tree.

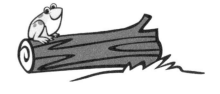

My Kindergarten Reading Workbook

98. A Trip to the Store

Read the story. Then answer each question by coloring the correct picture.

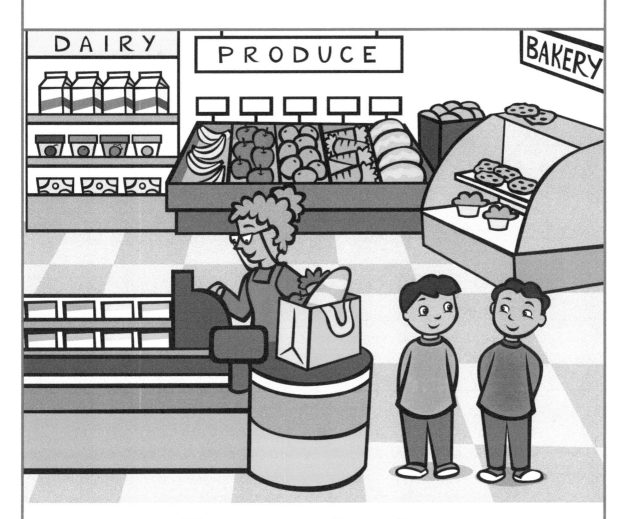

A Trip to the Store

We go to the store. We get some fruit. We need some milk.
Look at the cookies! We buy 2 cookies! We pay and leave.

Who goes to the store?

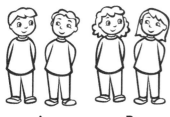

A.   B.

What do they get?

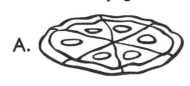

A.

B.

How many cookies do they buy?

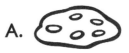

A.

B.

99. Good Night, Bear

Read the story. Circle the correct answer to each question.

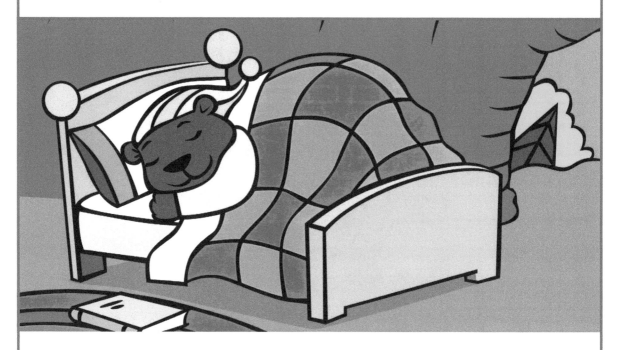

Good Night, Bear

Bear is tired. He is in a cave. He likes to read before bed. He gets his blanket. He shuts his eyes. Good night, Bear!

Questions

1. How does Bear feel?

A. happy   B. tired   C. sad

2. What does Bear get before he shuts his eyes?

A. a toy   B. a drink   C. a blanket

3. Where is Bear?

A. a cave   B. a house   C. a tent

4. What does Bear do last in the story?

A. gets into bed   B. reads a book   C. shuts his eyes

My Kindergarten Reading Workbook

100. Sand Search

Read the sentences. Then find and color the objects in the sentences.

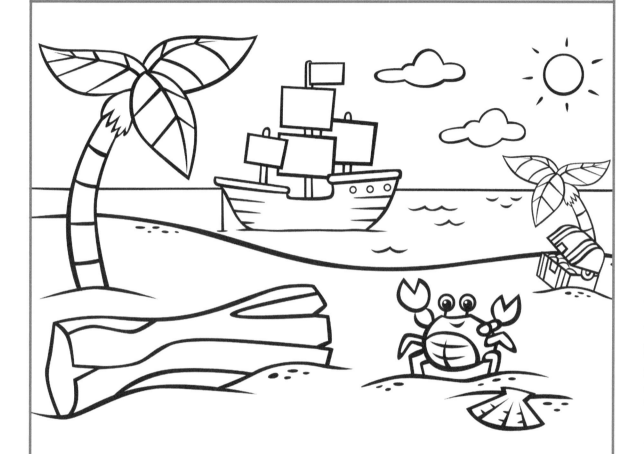

I see a big tree.

Do you see the shell?

I like the ship.

The sun is bright.

101. Where Am I?

Read each clue. Then draw a line to the matching place.

We wash dishes and set
the table.

farm

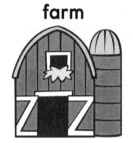

I see a barn and cows
in the field.

library

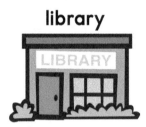

There are books on the shelf
that we can borrow.

kitchen

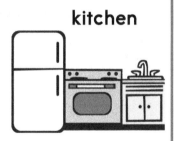

I like to sit in the grass.
I like to play tag.

school

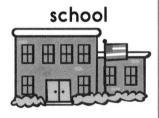

My teacher is nice.
We learn new things.

park

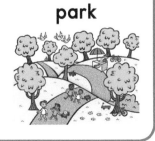

My Kindergarten Reading Workbook

Answer Key

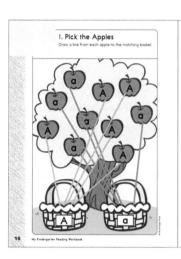

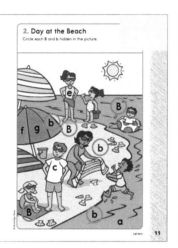

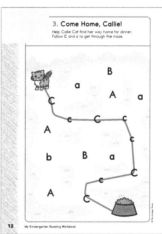

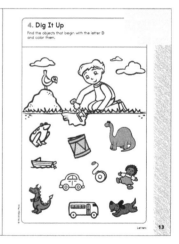

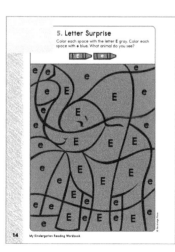

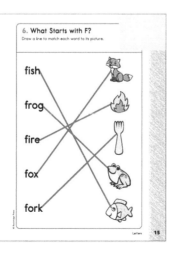

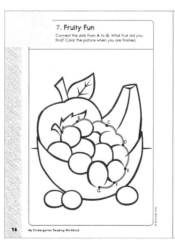

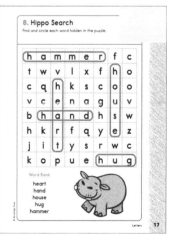

9. Ice Cream for Izzy
Izzy Penguin wants an ice cream cone! Follow I and i to help her through the maze.

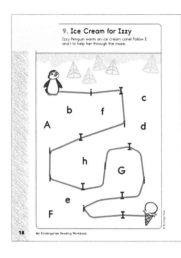

10. In the Jungle
Circle each J and j hidden in the picture.

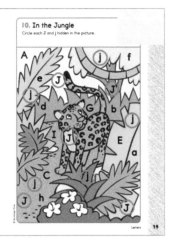

11. Fly a Kite
Color the picture below to fly a kite. Color the K spaces blue and the k spaces red.

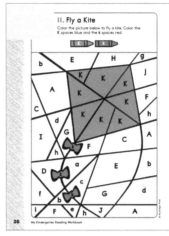

12. Look for Ll
Get 3 in a row by circling the pictures that begin with the letter Ll.

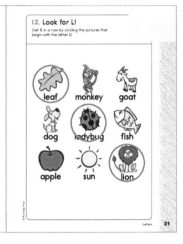

13. Hang Around
Help Mia Monkey fill in the missing letters in the crossword puzzle.

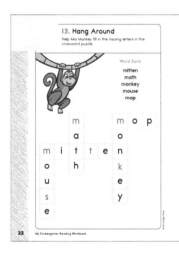

14. Build a Nest
Connect the dots from A to N to make a nest! Say each letter out loud as you connect it. Color the picture when you are finished.

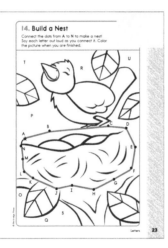

15. Out of this World
Ollie Alien is looking for objects that start with the letter O. Find and circle each one.

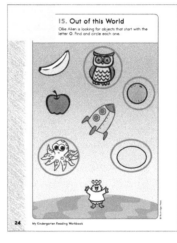

16. P is for . . .
Color the pictures that begin with the letter P! Can you get 3 in a row?

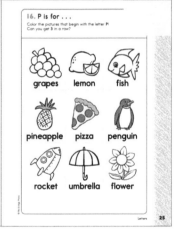

17. Castle Quest
Follow Q and q to help the knight get to the castle!

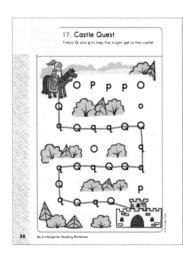

18. In My Room
Find and circle each object that begins with the letter R.

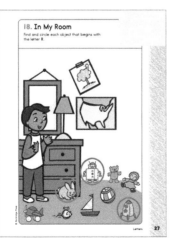

19. Silly Scramble
Unscramble the letters and write each word. The pictures will give you a hint.

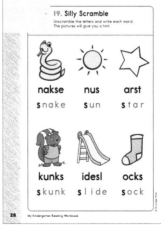

nakse — snake   nus — sun   arst — star

kunks — skunk   idesl — slide   ocks — sock

20. Time to Camp
The stars are shining! Draw a line from each T and t to the matching tent.

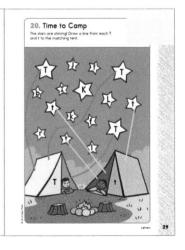

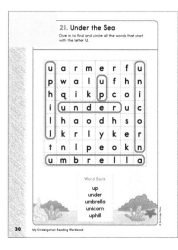

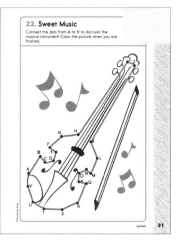

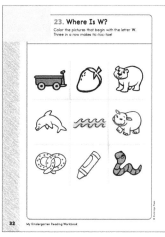

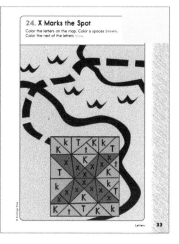

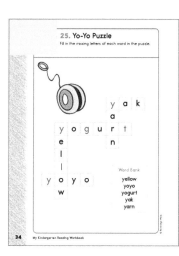

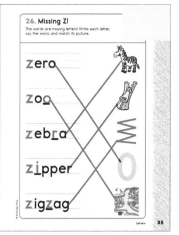

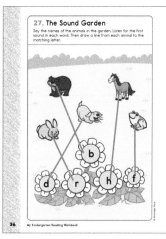

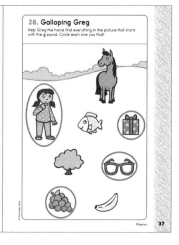

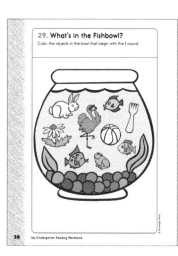

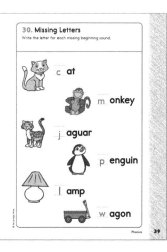

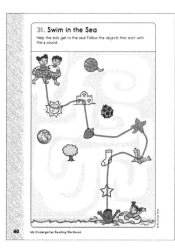

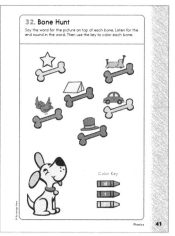

33. Match the Ends
Say the name of each picture. Listen for the end sound in the word. Then draw a line from the picture to the sound.

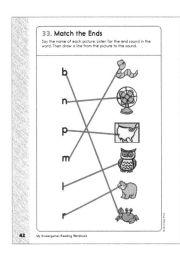

34. Brett in the Boat
Help Brett Bear fish for objects. Circle each one that ends with the t sound!

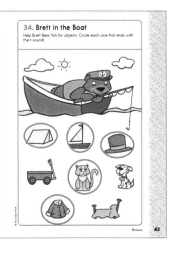

35. Listen for X!
Which objects end with the letter X? Find and color each one to get 3 in a row!

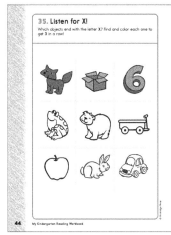

36. What Is Missing?
The sounds are missing from the ends of the words! Write the letter of each missing sound.

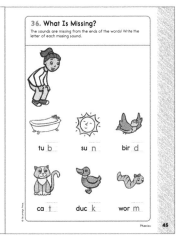

tu b   su n   bir d

ca t   duc k   wor m

37. Choo Choo!
Say each word in the puzzle. Do you hear the short a sound? Or do you hear the long a sound? Listen and then use the guide to color the picture.

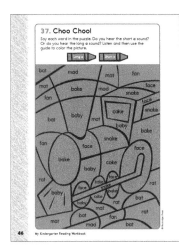

38. Lost in Space
Help Andy Astronaut find the long and short a words in the puzzle.

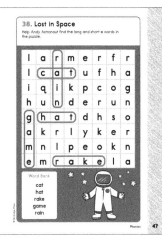

39. Listen for the Long Sound!
Color the pictures that have a long e sound. Three in a row makes tic-tac-toe!

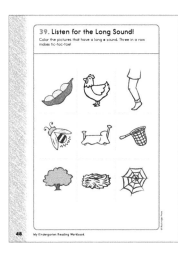

40. Web of Words
Can you finish the crossword? Use the picture clues to help you fill in the puzzle. The words contain the long and short e sounds.

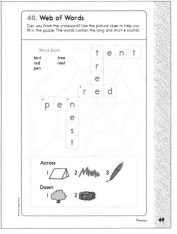

41. Short Surprise
Start at the star and draw a line to connect the dots. Say the word at each dot. Can you hear the short i sound? Color the picture when you are finished.

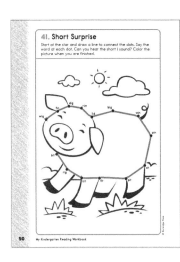

42. Ice Cream Shop
Circle the ice cream cones with words that have the long i sound.

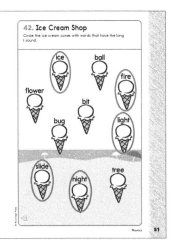

43. Climb Up the Tree
Help Otto get to his tree house! Follow the words with a short o sound to get through the maze.

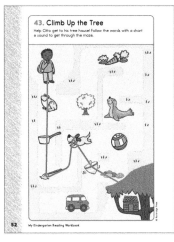

44. Snow Search
Use the picture clues to fill in the crossword puzzle. Each word has the long o sound.

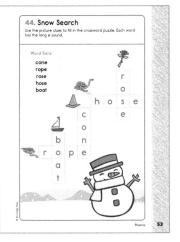

114   Answer Key

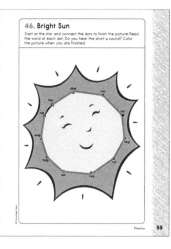

45. Unicorn Puzzle
Find and circle each word with a long u sound.

j	a	r	m	c	u	b	e
u	c	a	t	u	f	h	a
i	t	i	k	p	l	o	i
c	u	n	d	e	u	u	n
e	b	a	t	d	t	s	o
a	e	r	l	y	e	e	r
m	n	l	p	e	o	k	n
e	g	l	u	e	v	l	a

Word Bank
cube
glue
tube
flute
juice

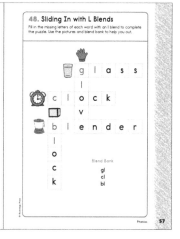

46. Bright Sun
Start at the star and connect the dots to finish the picture! Read the word at each dot. Do you hear the short u sound? Color the picture when you are finished.

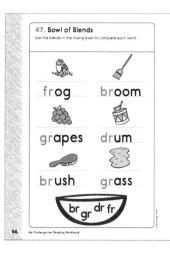

47. Bowl of Blends
Use the blends in the mixing bowl to complete each word.

frog   broom

grapes   drum

brush   grass

br gr dr fr

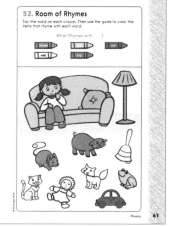

48. Sliding In with L Blends
Fill in the missing letters of each word with an l blend to complete the puzzle. Use the pictures and blend bank to help you out.

g l a s s
c l o c k
b l e n d e r

Blend Bank
gl
cl
bl

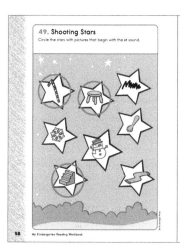

49. Shooting Stars
Circle the stars with pictures that begin with the st sound.

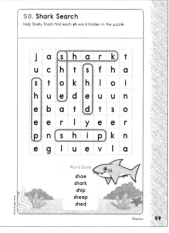

50. Shark Search
Help Shelly Shark find each sh word hidden in the puzzle.

j	a	s	h	a	r	k	t
u	c	h	t	s	f	h	a
s	t	o	k	h	l	o	i
h	u	e	d	e	u	u	n
e	b	a	t	d	t	s	o
e	e	r	l	y	e	e	r
p	n	s	h	i	p	k	n
e	g	l	u	e	v	l	a

Word Bank
shoe
shark
ship
sheep
shed

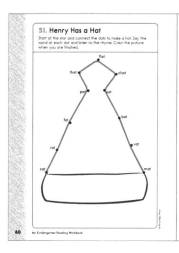

51. Henry Has a Hat
Start at the star and connect the dots to make a hat. Say the word at each dot and listen to the rhyme. Color the picture when you are finished.

flat
that   chat
pat   sat
fat   bat
rat   vat
cat   mat

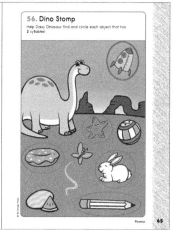

52. Room of Rhymes
Say the word on each crayon. Then use the guide to color the items that rhyme with each word.

What Rhymes with . . . ?

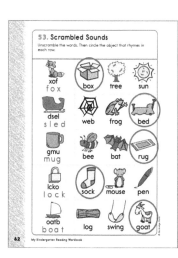

53. Scrambled Sounds
Unscramble the words. Then circle the object that rhymes in each row.

xof
f o x   box   tree   sun

dsel
s l e d   web   frog   bed

gmu
m u g   bee   bat   rug

lcko
l o c k   sock   mouse   pen

oatb
b o a t   log   swing   goat

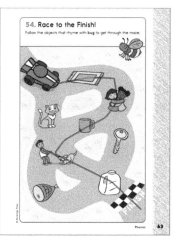

54. Race to the Finish!
Follow the objects that rhyme with bug to get through the maze.

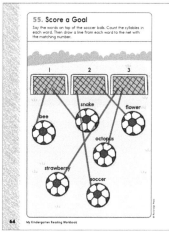

55. Score a Goal
Say the words on top of the soccer balls. Count the syllables in each word. Then draw a line from each word to the net with the matching number.

1   2   3

bee   snake   flower
octopus
strawberry
soccer

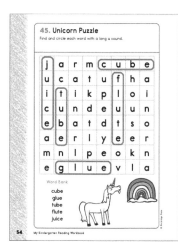

56. Dino Stomp
Help Daisy Dinosaur find and circle each object that has 2 syllables!

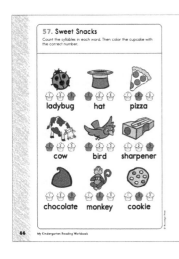

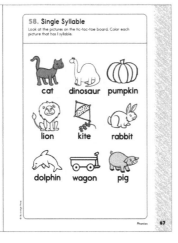

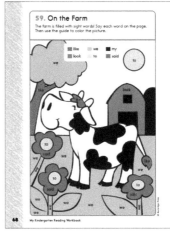

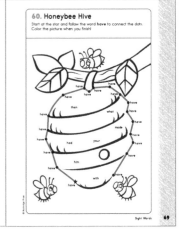

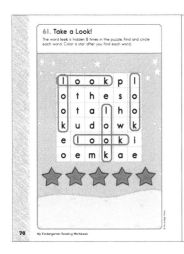

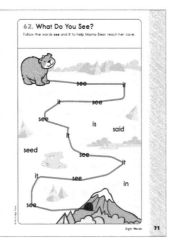

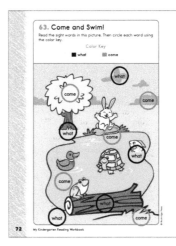

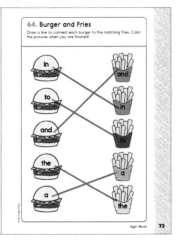

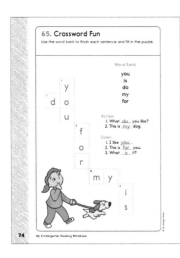

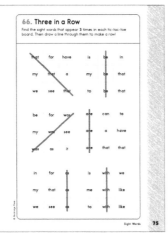

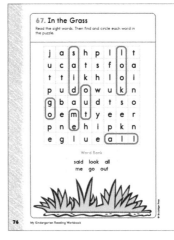

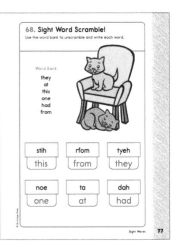

116   Answer Key

69. In the Ocean
Color the fish using the color key.

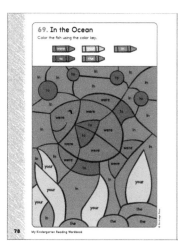

70. Down the Hill
Can you find the sight words in this puzzle? Be sure to look across and down.

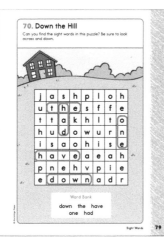

71. I Can Fly!
Help the bird fly back to her nest! Follow and trace the word can to get through the maze.

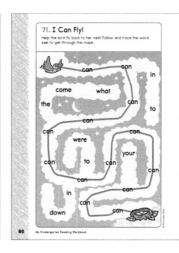

72. Crunchy Apples
Read the sight word on each apple. Find the basket with the matching word. Draw a line to connect each apple with the correct basket.

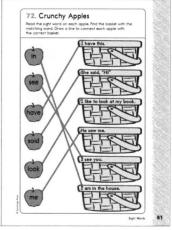

73. Read and Write Sight Words
Use the word bank to find the missing word in each sentence. Then write the correct words to finish the puzzle.

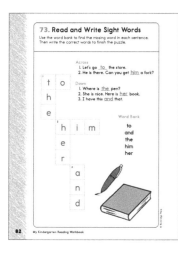

74. Time for Tic-Tac-Toe
Draw a line through the sight words that appear 3 times in each tic-tac-toe board. Three in a row wins!

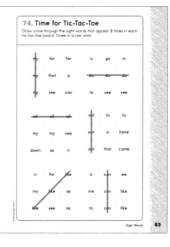

75. The Wishing Well
Find and circle each sight word in the puzzle. Be sure to look across and down. Make a wish when you finish!

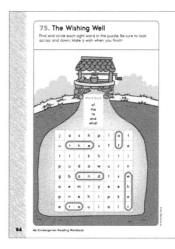

76. Jumbled Up
Unscramble and write each word. Use the word bank to help you.

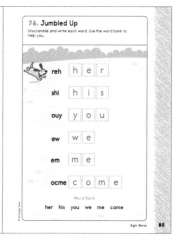

77. Fish Tank Fun
Color each fish in the tank using the color key.

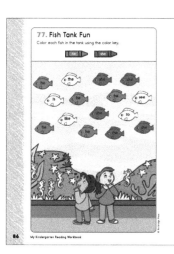

78. Strike Out Sight Words
Put an X over the sight words that appear 3 times in each tic-tac-toe board.

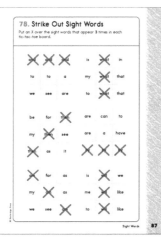

79. A Sunny Day
Start at the star. Connect the dots and say each sight word out loud to finish the sentence. What do you see when you connect the dots? Color the picture when you are finished.

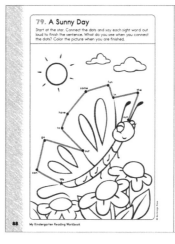

80. Milk and Cookies
Time for a snack! Start at the milk carton and color the boxes with the word said to get to the cookie. YUM!

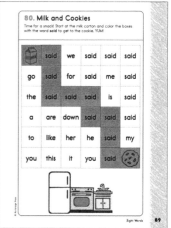

Answer Key   **117**

81. Up, Up, and Away
Read the words in the balloons. Then draw lines to connect the matching balloons. Color the pictures when you are finished.

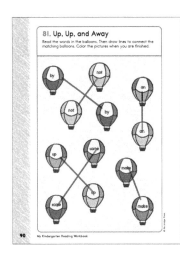

82. Clown Around
Can you solve the crossword? Use the word bank to find the missing word in each sentence.

Across
1. The apple is good.
2. I can do it!

Down
1. How are you?
2. I fell down.
3. This is big.

Word Bank
how
good
this
down
can

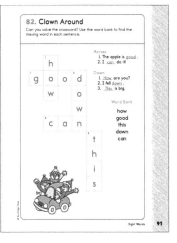

83. Castle Search
Find and circle each word in the puzzle!

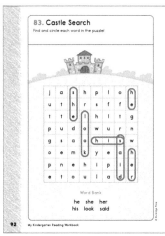

Word Bank
he she her
his look said

84. Where Is the Bird?
Circle the words that match each picture.

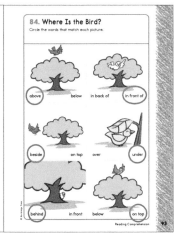

85. Leo Lion
Read the sentences below. Then draw a line to match each sentence to its picture.

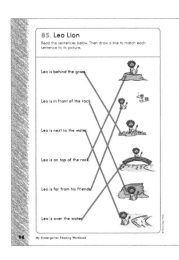

86. Color the Pairs
Read the words on the page. Find and color each pair of opposite words. Use the same color for each opposite pair.

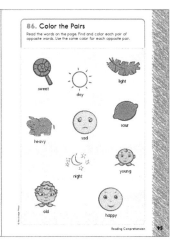

87. Matching Opposites
Read each word in the left column. Then draw a line to the opposite word in the right column.

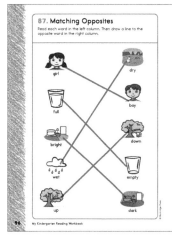

88. Scrambled-Up Opposites
Read each word on the left. Then unscramble and write the word in each opposite pair.

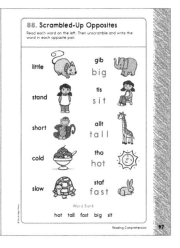

little — gib → **big**
stand — tis → **sit**
short — allt → **tall**
cold — tho → **hot**
slow — staf → **fast**

Word Bank
hot tall fast big sit

89. A Day at the Park
Read each action word. Then find and circle the matching part of the picture.

Word Bank
hop
throw
read
eat
drive
paint

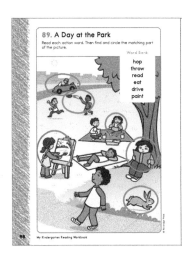

90. Mixed-Up Words
Unscramble and write each action word. Use the word bank and pictures to help you.

Word Bank
jump run swim climb fly

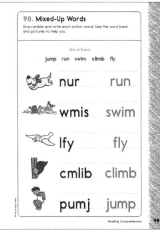

nur — **run**
wmis — **swim**
lfy — **fly**
cmlib — **climb**
pumj — **jump**

91. Action Tic-Tac-Toe!
Read the sentences in each tic-tac-toe square. Put an X on each sentence that has an action word in it. Can you find 3 in a row?

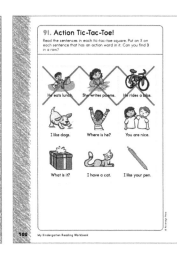

He eats lunch.   She writes poems.   He rides a bike.
I like dogs.   Where is he?   You are nice.
What is it?   I have a cat.   I like your pen.

92. The Dog
Read the story. Then circle the answer to each question below.

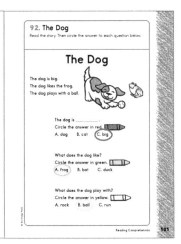

The Dog

The dog is big.
The dog likes the frog.
The dog plays with a ball.

The dog is __
Circle the answer in red.
A. dog   B. cat   **C. big**

What does the dog like?
Circle the answer in green.
A. frog   B. bat   C. duck

What does the dog play with?
Circle the answer in yellow.
A. rock   **B. ball**   C. run

93. My Messy Desk
Read the sentences. Then color the picture to match each sentence.

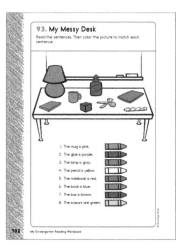

1. The rug is pink.
2. The glue is purple.
3. The lamp is gray.
4. The pencil is yellow.
5. The notebook is red.
6. The book is blue.
7. The box is brown.
8. The scissors are green.

94. My Day
Read the story. Then unscramble and write the words from the story.

My Day

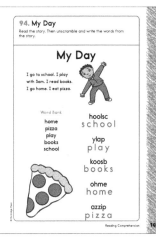

I go to school. I play
with Sam. I read books.
I go home. I eat pizza.

Word Bank
home
pizza
play
books
school

hoolsc s c h o o l

ylap p l a y

koosb b o o k s

ohme h o m e

azzip p i z z a

95. Fruit Bowl Fun!
Read the story. Then choose 3 questions in the tic-tac-toe board. Answer and circle 3 questions in a row to win!

Answers will vary.

My Fruit Bowl

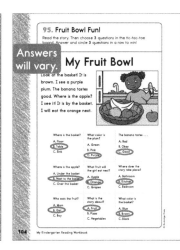

Look at the basket! It is
brown. I see a purple
plum. The banana tastes
good. Where is the apple?
I see it! It is by the basket.
I will eat the orange next.

Where is the basket?	What color is the plum?	The banana tastes . . .
A. Floor	A. Green	A. Bad
B. Table	B. Pink	B. Okay
C. Sink	C. Purple	C. Good

Where is the apple?	What fruit will the girl eat next?	Where does the story take place?
A. Under the basket	A. Apple	A. Bathroom
B. Next to the basket	B. Orange	B. Kitchen
C. Over the basket	C. Grapes	C. Bedroom

Who eats the fruit?	What is the story about?	What color is the basket?
A. Mom	A. Fruit	A. Blue
B. Girl	B. Pizza	B. Brown
C. Boy	C. Vegetables	C. Black

96. A Day at the Farm
Read the story. Then color the animals that were in the story.

A Day at the Farm

I am at the farm. I see many things. There is a cow.
There are pigs. Over there is a horse. I like the chickens.

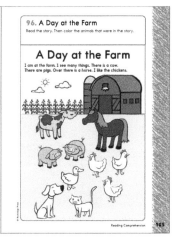

97. Read and Match
Draw a line from each sentence to the matching picture.

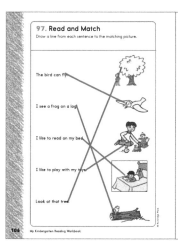

The bird can fly.

I see a frog on a log.

I like to read on my bed.

I like to play with my toys.

Look at that tree.

98. A Trip to the Store
Read the story. Then answer each question by coloring the correct picture.

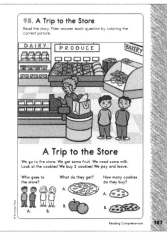

A Trip to the Store

We go to the store. We get some fruit. We need some milk.
Look at the cookies! We buy 2 cookies! We pay and leave.

Who goes to the store? / What do they get? / How many cookies do they buy?

99. Good Night, Bear
Read the story. Circle the correct answer to each question.

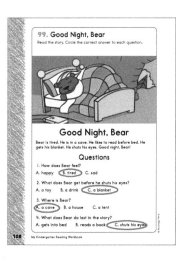

Good Night, Bear

Bear is tired. He is in a cave. He likes to read before bed. He
gets his blanket. He shuts his eyes. Good night, Bear!

Questions
1. How does Bear feel?
   A. happy   B. tired   C. sad
2. What does Bear get before he shuts his eyes?
   A. a toy   B. a drink   C. a blanket
3. Where is Bear?
   A. a cave   B. a house   C. a tent
4. What does Bear do last in the story?
   A. gets into bed   B. reads a book   C. shuts his eyes

100. Sand Search
Read the sentences. Then find and color the objects in the sentences.

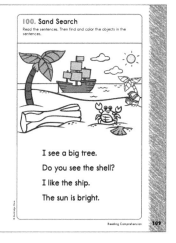

I see a big tree.

Do you see the shell?

I like the ship.

The sun is bright.

101. Where Am I?
Read each clue. Then draw a line to the matching place.

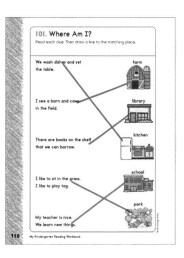

We wash dishes and set the table.   — farm

I see a barn and cows in the field.   — library

There are books on the shelf that we can borrow.   — kitchen

I like to sit in the grass. I like to play tag.   — school

My teacher is nice. We learn new things.   — park

Answer Key   **119**

About the Author

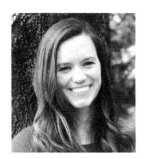 **KIMBERLY ANN KIEDROWSKI** is a former kindergarten teacher of almost 10 years. She creates resources for teachers to use in their classrooms and loves to share her teaching ideas on her blog (www.LiveLaughILoveKindergarten.com). Kim holds a bachelor of science degree in early childhood education from the University of Wisconsin-Green Bay. When she is not blogging or creating, she is spending time with her husband and kids.

YOU DID IT!

You are on the fast track to reading!

_____

(your name)

has completed all the activities in

My Kindergarten Reading Workbook.

Reading is fun!

Continue the Learning Fun!

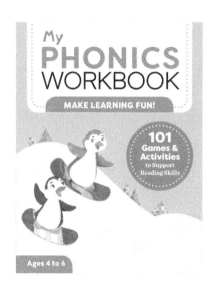

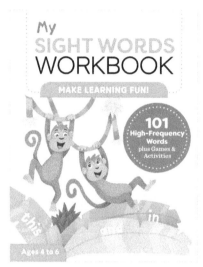

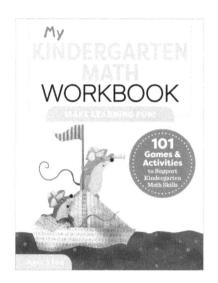

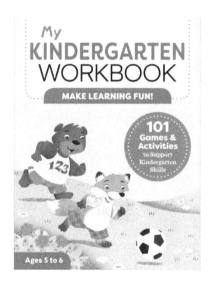

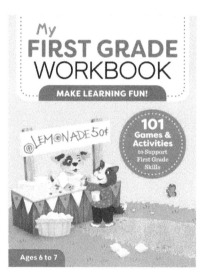

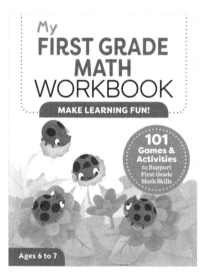

ROCKRIDGE
PRESS

Available wherever books are sold.

CPSIA information can be obtained
at www.ICGtesting.com
Printed in the USA
JSHW011908200621
16049JS00001B/1